Eating Disorders and Weight Loss Research

EATING DISORDERS AND WEIGHT LOSS RESEARCH

JEROME S. RUBIN
EDITOR

Nova Science Publishers, Inc.
New York

For permission to use material from this book please contact us:
Telephone 631-231-7269; Fax 631-231-8175
Web Site: http://www.novapublishers.com

Library of Congress Cataloging-in-Publication Data

Eating disorders and weight loss research / Jerome S. Rubin (editor).
p. ; cm.
Includes bibliographical references and index.
ISBN 1-60021-334-0
1. Eating disorders. 2. Weight loss. I. Rubin, Jerome S., 1964-
[DNLM: 1. Eating Disorders. 2. Diet. 3. Eating. 4. Weight Loss. WM 175 E14619 2006]
RC552.E18.E282114 2006
616.85'26--dc22 2006021083

Published by Nova Science Publishers, Inc. ✣New York

CONTENTS

PREFACE

The abundance of food in the developed countries of the world has seemingly spawned an epidemic of disorders connected to the food. Extremes such as intensive concern about one's body image and total disregard for it have resulted in countries which contain enormous segments of the population who are either obese or bordering on anorexia nervosa. This new book gathers state-of-the-art research from leading scientists throughout the world which offers important information on understanding the underlying causes and discovering the most effective treatments for eating disorders.

Chapter 1 - A substantial gap exists between scientific evidence and clinical practice in the psychological treatment of eating disorders. Not only are eating disorders commonly described as addictions by laypersons and mental health professionals alike, but surveys indicate that approximately one-third of eating disorder treatment programs and clinicians use addictions-based psychotherapies to treat eating disorders. However, the validity of the addiction model of eating disorders has received little empirical study and the efficacy of addictions-based psychotherapies for eating disorders remains untested. Understanding the extent of association between eating disorders and addictions has important implications for treatment, prevention, and our understanding of the etiology of eating disorders. This chapter examines issues surrounding the definition of addiction, reviews theoretical reasoning and empirical evidence regarding the addiction model of eating disorders, discusses the construct of "addictive disorder" and identifies future research directions.

Chapter 2 - Various biological, psychological, and sociocultural factors have been considered in the attempt to understand the etiology of eating pathologies such as anorexia nervosa and bulimia nervosa. Psychosexual issues are neither sufficient nor necessary for the development of an eating disorder in a young person, and it should be considered as only one factor in the multidimensional, multifactorial framework needed to clarify this complex and still poorly understood set of disorders. In particular, gender roles and sociocultural expectations appear strongly implicated in the development of eating disorders, since anorexia nervosa and bulimia nervosa occur predominantly among women. This is frequently attributed to the continued emphasis on physical attractiveness and a thin physique for women. In consequence, women reportedly express greater dissatisfaction about their bodies, more concern with appearance and body weight, and more frequently engage in weight-control efforts. Since at least 90 per cent of eating disordered patients are females, then it would therefore seem plausible to suggest that the female role might play a part in the genesis of these pathologies. This fact strongly supports that the meaning of femininity in Western society has some relationship with the development of eating. Eating disorders are common, serious illnesses that present major challenges to physicians and other health care professionals. Sociocultural body norms for ideal size and shape may be reinforced by participation in activities, sports, or membership in groups that promotes weight loss and shape change. Eating disorders are furthermore reinforced when high status individuals (e.g. parents, teachers, coaches, doctors) encourage a susceptible individual to diet. Studies indicate that a complex combination of genetic and sociocultural-developmental factors is responsible for the onset of these illnesses.

Chapter 3 - Eating disorders are today an increasing problem among teenagers and young adults specially females. In the case of bulimia the estimated prevalence is between 3 and 5% and the average age it starts is around 20 years. It is known that its etiology is complex and depends on biological, psychological, and social factors as well as more specific characteristics as, for example, the practice of sports that in some cases leads to these disorders. The close relation between corporal image and performance makes the female athletes a group particularly vulnerable to problems of bulimic behavior due to the emphasis in weight control that they are frequently submitted. However the studies available are still insufficient to characterize the amplitude and distribution of the problem. The aim of the present work is to evaluate bulimic components of behavior among adolescent female endurance runners. From a total of 40 athletes affiliated with the Track and Field Federation of Rio de Janeiro, 17 female endurance runners (16 ± 1.8 years old) and 32 post-menarche, non-athletic adolescents (15.0 ± 1.4 years) were examined. The athletes were training for at least 2 years (15 ± 7 hours/week). The body composition was esteemed by the anthropometric method and percent body fat (%F) and Body Mass Index (BMI) were calculated. Bulimic behavioral components (frequency and severity) were evaluated using the Portuguese version of BITE (Bulimic Investigatory Test, Edinburgh), a self-rating scale. A control group of 32 non-athlete volunteers in the same age group were also evaluated. Calculation of parameters, descriptive data statistics and comparison (Anova one way) of the variables were performed with the software Statistica for windows (5.1, 1998), with a significant level of $p \leq 0,05$. Scores above the normal limit of 10 were recorded for 35.3% of the athletes (6 individuals), including 29.4% (4 individuals) that reported unusual behavioral components, suggestive of a tendency toward bulimia. One individual scored above 20, indicating a possible clinical case of bulimia. On the scale of severity of the symptoms, a score of 5 (considered moderately severe) was recorded in one case. The athletes in this group are in risk to develop eating disorder, considering their preoccupation with weight control and the use of inadequate means of keeping within the desired range – including restrictive practices such as fasting along with intense physical activity.

Chapter 4 - Rumination is the regurgitation of recently ingested food and is one of the most commonly occurring eating disorders in persons with developmental disabilities. Rumination might result in the negative side effect of foul breath and can interfere with a person's opportunities to engage in social interactions. Additionally, medical side effects include weight loss, aspiration pneumonia, and tooth decay. The published research studies that examined the efficacy of behavioral-intervention packages to reduce rumination are summarized in this chapter. This chapter also reviews the clinical effectiveness and generality of these intervention packages and highlights recent clinical advancements in the treatment of rumination.

Chapter 5 - Patients with eating disorders (EDs) are secretive with regard to their eating behaviors, and clinicians often experience difficulty in assessing their status using interviews or self-reported questionnaires. Although evaluations of clinical status should be made during treatment, few biological markers of eating behaviors in patients with anorexia nervosa and bulimia nervosa have been identified. Thus, the development of more useful markers is required in order to ensure successful treatment. In previous research on EDs, carbohydrate metabolism appeared to be associated with nutritional status; however, carbohydrate markers with which to assess eating behaviors remained to be identified. This chapter explores the relationship between carbohydrate metabolism and eating behaviors in these patients, and presents recent research on a new carbohydrate marker, the insulinogenic index at 15 minutes, which precisely mirrors eating behaviors in patients with EDs. The authors also address the clinical significance of assessing eating behaviors in patients with EDs from the biological perspective and discuss future directions in the field.

Chapter 6 - It is well recognized that the prevalence of metabolic abnormalities found in the presence of obesity is increasing within our sedentary population. In fact, obesity is a growing epidemic that is primarily due to environmental influences. There has been a rapid increase in obesity over the past 30 years in North America, whereas the recent prevalence estimations from self-reported data in Canada indicated that 15 % of the adult population is obese and 33 % is classified in the overweight category, while in the US nearly 1/3 of adults are obese, corresponding to almost 20 % of the US population [1-3]. This highlights the importance of environmental factors and lifestyle choices since obesity cannot be totally explained by genetic factors alone [4]. Unfortunately, sedentary lifestyle and increased energy intake predispose to high fat and high calorie food choices, and refined diet seems to be adopted by an increasing proportion of our population. This is leading to weight gain, positive energy balance, obesity and health-related complications. Thus, "at risk" obesity (abdominal obesity) is an important cause of metabolic complications, such as cardiovascular disease (CVD), type 2 diabetes, hypertension, and the metabolic syndrome (MetS) [5-7]. Indeed, the American Heart Association (AHA) has classified obesity as a modifiable risk factor for coronary heart disease (CHD) [8]. A variety of therapies may help to reduce the incidence of obesity and the MetS, including diet, physical exercise, and pharmacological treatments. Weight loss is an essential component in the management of the metabolic complications of obesity as well as the MetS itself. Low-fat diets have been advocated for weight loss for many years. However, some popular diets such as the very low-carbohydrate (ketogenic) diets have challenged the effectiveness of conventional low-fat diets, partly because of there rapid efficiency in contrast to the continuing increased prevalence of obesity despite reductions of fat intake. Thus, several authors have compared the effectiveness of various weight loss approaches, such as those proposed by the official guidelines, to the "popular" diets (as Atkins, Ornish, The Zone, South Beach diet, Weight Watchers) in the management of obesity and its related complications. Although, there is a need to perform well designed clinical trials showing long-term safety and efficacy of low-carbohydrate diets, several studies have showed effective short-term weight loss and improved metabolic characteristics of the MetS compared to low-fat diets. The major targets of intervention for proper treatment of the epidemic of obesity remain weight loss and active lifestyle. Even if different types of diet or diet/exercise combinations can produce weight loss; if this treatment is stopped, weight is regained. The current review underlines the clinical and the experimental evidence of the different dietary approaches for weight loss regarding obesity treatment and related metabolic complications. Despite numerous researches, there is still controversy regarding the optimal macronutrient content, and we also overview the issue of carbohydrate restriction versus fat restriction on weight loss and weight control in order to achieve effective weight loss and better health. Indeed, modest weight reduction (5 % to 10 % of body weight) can decrease total cholesterol, improve glucose tolerance and decrease blood pressure in overweight and type 2 diabetic patients [6;9-12]. This review also discusses the consequences of obesity management on the MetS, which represents a cluster of several specific metabolic abnormalities recognized to increase CVD, type 2 diabetes and cardiovascular mortality [6;7;13]. Considering that recent prospective studies show that obesity seems to be the central component of the MetS [5;6], and epidemiological studies have showed that these high-risk individuals have a three-fold increment in CVD and cardiovascular mortality, weight loss is recommended as a first-line therapy [7;14;15]. We also briefly discuss the role of several dietary interventions, which can lower CHD risk and improve lipid profile.

In: Eating Disorders and Weight Loss Research
Editor: Jerome S. Rubin, pp. 1-37
ISBN 1-60021-1-334-0

Chapter 1

Eating Disorders and Addiction: Theory and Evidence

Kristin M. von Ranson and Stephanie E. Cassin
Department of Psychology, University of Calgary, Canada

Abstract

A substantial gap exists between scientific evidence and clinical practice in the psychological treatment of eating disorders. Not only are eating disorders commonly described as addictions by laypersons and mental health professionals alike, but surveys indicate that approximately one-third of eating disorder treatment programs and clinicians use addictions-based psychotherapies to treat eating disorders. However, the validity of the addiction model of eating disorders has received little empirical study and the efficacy of addictions-based psychotherapies for eating disorders remains untested. Understanding the extent of association between eating disorders and addictions has important implications for treatment, prevention, and our understanding of the etiology of eating disorders. This chapter examines issues surrounding the definition of addiction, reviews theoretical reasoning and empirical evidence regarding the addiction model of eating disorders, discusses the construct of "addictive disorder" and identifies future research directions.

Introduction

A large, sometimes conflicting literature on associations between eating disorders and addictions—sometimes also termed addictive behaviors or disorders—has developed in recent years. A number of reviews of the conceptualization of eating disorders as forms of addiction have been prepared (e.g., Bemis, 1985; Vandereycken, 1990; Wilson, 1991; Wilson, 1993; Wilson, 1999; Wilson, 2000, 2002; Wilson and Latner, 2001). After critically examining empirical and theoretical support for the "addiction model" of eating disorders,[1]

[1] Although mention is made here and elsewhere in the literature of an "addiction model" of eating disorders as if there were only one, in fact there are variations, as is discussed later in this chapter. These addiction models

these reviews have generally concluded that neither convincing empirical support nor sound theoretical basis exists for conceiving of eating disorders as addictions. To many researchers, it is a given that conceiving of or treating eating disorders as addictions is unfounded. It is striking, however, that others persistently contend that addictions-based treatment approaches for eating disorders have merit. For example, clinicians have adapted psychotherapeutic strategies from existing addictions treatments for individuals with eating disorders (e.g., Johnson and Sansone, 1993; Johnson and Taylor, 1996; McAleavey and Fiumara, 2001; Riley, 1991; Trotzky, 2002; Weiner, 1998). This ongoing contradiction between research-based recommendations and actual clinical practice suggests a need to carefully re-examine the topic of the addiction model of eating disorders.

Despite a great deal of empirical interest in certain questions related to the addiction model of eating disorders, such as the degree to which eating disorders co-occur with such core addictions as substance abuse, many facets of this model remain unexamined. The dearth of empirical investigation into many aspects of the addiction model of eating disorders may have resulted in part from to the absence of systematic information on the frequency of use of addictions-based approaches in the treatment of eating disorders. In other words, it has not been clear in practical terms just how significant an issue the addiction model of eating disorders really is. Until recently, no published studies described the frequency of use of addictions-based approaches. However, results of a recent telephone survey demonstrated that more than a quarter (26.9%) of psychotherapists in a large Canadian city who regularly provided services to individuals with eating disorders often or always folded addictions-based approaches into their eating disorder treatment, and an additional 15.4% of psychotherapists referred clients to adjunctive addictions-based treatments (von Ranson and Robinson, 2006). Thus, a substantial minority (42.3%) of these psychotherapists either used or promoted services with addictions-based eating disorder treatments, indicating that some form of the addiction model of eating disorders is widely embraced by clinical practitioners.

It would be time-consuming and quite challenging—probably prohibitively so—to determine the psychotherapeutic orientations of treatment programs that treat individuals with eating disorders, particularly those available across a wide range of locations. However, the advent of the internet provides an opportunity to describe those treatment programs that have websites. Between October and December 2004, we conducted a systematic survey of English-language internet websites advertising or describing treatment services emphasizing eating disorders to determine what proportion included an addictions component.[2] This survey identified 177 eating disorder treatment program sites; of these programs, 54 (30.5%) used an addictions-based approach, including 12-step programs, as part or the entirety of their treatment of an eating disorder. Addictions-based treatment programs were located primarily across the United States (87.0%), but sites were also identified in Canada (5.6%), the United

have in common an emphasis on the apparent addictive nature of eating disorder symptoms. For simplicity, we use the term "addiction model" in this chapter to refer to those theories or views of eating disorders that focus on the centrality of addictive elements in the etiology of the eating disorder, its maintenance, or both.

[2] The search engine used was www.google.ca. Search terms included combinations of "eating disorder," "anorexia," and "bulimia" with "treatment," "addiction," and "12-step." As search results yielded very large numbers of hits (e.g., > 2,620,000) and later results tended to be repetitions of previously visited sites or sites that yielded no additional information, not all search results were examined. Instead, the first 100 "eating disorder treatment" websites were examined as well as the first 50 results from the remaining searches. Websites were excluded from this analysis if (1) they were written in a language other than English or (2) did not mention

Kingdom (5.6%), and South Africa (1.9%). Although the eating disorder treatment websites identified are unlikely to constitute a representative sample of eating disorder treatment programs in these locations, it is important to note that the present internet-based findings are quite consistent with those found in the telephone survey described above, which described the psychotherapeutic orientation of psychotherapists in Calgary, Canada (von Ranson and Robinson, 2006). Taken together, these survey findings suggest that addictions-based treatment approaches for eating disorders are widespread across North America and are used by approximately one-third of eating disorder treatment programs and practitioners.

Consistent with findings of professional psychotherapeutic approaches offered, eating disorders are also commonly considered addictions by laypersons. Addictions-based self-help treatments for eating disorders, most prominently Overeaters Anonymous (e.g., Ronel and Libman, 2003), are commonplace across North America. We describe and discuss the tenets of Overeaters Anonymous in detail later in this chapter.

Another important reason to study the validity of the addiction model of eating disorders is that implications for treatment vary dramatically according to differing etiological and conceptual models of eating disorders. For example, cognitive behavioral therapy, widely accepted as the most efficacious treatment for bulimia nervosa (e.g., Fairburn, 2002; Thompson-Brenner, Glass, and Westen, 2003; Wilson and Pike, 2001), is based on a model that emphasizes the role of both cognitive and behavioral factors in the maintenance of eating disorders. The *cognitive-behavioral model* of bulimia nervosa asserts that when women overvalue weight and shape and restrict their food intake in order to achieve the sociocultural ideal of beauty, some become vulnerable to periodic loss of control over eating (Wilson and Pike, 2001). Purging and other compensatory behaviors are used to compensate for the effects of binge eating, but also help maintain binge eating by reducing anxiety about potential weight gain and disrupting learned satiety signals that regulate food intake, both of which contribute to future binge eating (Wilson and Pike, 2001). Cognitive-behavioral treatment of bulimia nervosa centers on reducing dietary restraint and maladaptive attitudes about the significance of weight and shape, establishing regular, nutritionally balanced meals, and introducing previously avoided foods into a more flexible diet (Wilson and Pike, 2001).

In contrast, a prominent *addiction model* of eating disorders asserts that "food addiction" results from a physiological, biochemical condition of the body that creates cravings for refined carbohydrates and other food substances (Sheppard, 1993), such that the patient depends on and is unable to control his or her intake of certain food substances (Haddock and Dill, 1999). Following from this model, treatment of food addiction requires highly structured eating patterns and absolute abstinence from specific "addictive" foods, such as white flour and sugar (Yeary, 1987). Note that treatment recommendations arising from the addiction model—e.g., avoidance of specific foods—are at odds from those arising from the cognitive-behavioral model, the treatment for bulimia nervosa that has the greatest degree of empirical support—e.g., moderation in all food intake.

This chapter reviews the theoretical underpinnings of the addiction model of eating disorders and examines the literature addressing the merits and demerits of considering eating disorders as forms of addiction, with the dual goals of identifying common ground for clinicians and researchers and identifying issues for future research to address. Empirical

---

eating disorders as one of six major problems treated, suggesting a lack of specialization in eating disorders treatment.

research has examined limited questions regarding associations of eating disorders and addictions; however, it remains unclear what, if anything, eating disorders and addictions truly have in common. We examine commonalities and dissimilarities of eating disorders and addictions to determine what further evidence is needed to determine the value—or lack thereof—of conceptualizing eating disorders as addictions, and examine issues including those related to definitions and terminology, psychiatric comorbidity, genetic and family history, and treatment implications. A compelling argument can be made that, ultimately, the value of drawing analogies between eating disorders and addictive disorders (or any other psychiatric disorder, for that matter) is determined by the degree to which it advances our understanding of the etiology and maintenance of eating disorders and contributes to the development of more effective prevention and treatment programs (Wilson, 1991). Hence, the utility of the addiction model of eating disorders is our primary emphasis in the present chapter.

Why are Eating Disorders Compared to Addictions?

Over the past several decades in which eating disorders have come under increased study, they have been frequently likened to addictions, specifically substance use disorders (Szmukler and Tantam, 1984; Vandereycken, 1990). Parallel arguments have been made to consider eating disorders variants of personality disorders, obsessive-compulsive disorder, and affective disorder, on the basis of similar phenomenology, frequent comorbidity, and family history (e.g., Bellodi et al., 2001; Hudson et al., 2003; Hudson, Pope, Jonas, and Yurgelun-Todd, 1983; Lilenfeld et al., 1998). Several commonalities between eating disorders and addictions have been noted, including the following (Davis and Claridge, 1998; Lacey, 1993; Vandereycken, 1990): First, patients with bulimia nervosa exhibit certain addiction-like behaviors and correlates (e.g., preoccupation with the substance, loss of control, craving). Second, they commonly abuse psychoactive substances. Third, high rates of substance abuse among relatives of patients with bulimia nervosa have been reported. Fourth, laboratory findings suggested that eating disorders, like addictions, might involve the endogenous opioid systems. Fifth, some have theorized that eating disorders and addictive disorders may share certain personality features, such as proneness toward impulsiveness. This chapter will address the empirical evidence for these observations.

Are Eating Disorders "Feminine" Addictions?

The social construction of mental disorder and addiction provides the basis for a feminist interpretation of the striking gender differences in rates of eating disorders and substance misuse. Some have observed that substance use problems and eating disorders are gendered disorders, in which eating disorders are prototypically "feminine" problems whereas substance use disorders are prototypically "masculine" problems (Reid and Burr, 2000). Eating disorders can be construed as a misguided attempt to impose control over the self, whereas substance use disorders can be viewed as involving a loss or abandonment of control. It is argued that women, who tend to have insufficient power and control in western society, may struggle to gain some control over their own bodies, resulting in an eating disorder in some, whereas men may have more power and responsibilities than they wish and try to escape through substance misuse (Reid and Burr, 2000). Although these ideas are intriguing, it is unclear how they might explain the tremendous range of individual responses to societal pressures related to masculinity and femininity, including why only some women develop an eating disorder and only some men develop substance misuse, and how some of both genders have neither problem or have both problems. Although admittedly methodologically challenging to study, it would be very interesting to integrate aspects of an approach that considers the meaning of mental disorder symptoms in evaluating empirically determined risk factors for eating disorders.

A Shared Biological Vulnerability?

A popular explanation for the association of eating disorders and psychoactive substance use disorders is that they result from a shared biological vulnerability (Jonas, 1990). The high rates of eating disorders in women and alcohol abuse in men have been hypothesized to be sex-specific expressions of an underlying "addictive" predisposition (e.g., Bulik, 1987). Societal constraints on excessive drinking by women have been theorized to make eating a more culturally available form of substance use and abuse (Bulik, 1987). Below we consider evidence addressing the hypothesis that a shared familial vulnerability toward addiction exists that may manifest differently across genders.

What is the Evidence for Comorbidity of Eating Disorders and Addictions?

Many have observed high rates of comorbidity of addictive behaviors with eating disorders. Substance use disorders (or "substance misuse") and compulsive gambling are recognized as major forms of addictions; although more controversial, some consider other repetitive behaviors—including compulsive sex, shopping, and internet use; kleptomania; fire-setting; trichotillomania; and intermittent explosive disorder—addictions as well (Holden, 2001). While little systematic research has examined whether eating disorders and pathological gambling are consistently linked, one study suggests they jointly occur (Lesieur and Blume, 1993). Individuals report gambling, eating, and using drugs for similar reasons, such as relief of anxiety, boredom, and depression (Lesieur and Blume, 1993). Research on "multi-impulsive personality disorder," theorized to affect a subset of individuals with bulimia nervosa who demonstrate a wide range of destructive, impulsive behaviors and have a poor prognosis, has examined the co-aggregation of various addictions in bulimic women (Lacey and Evans, 1986). A great deal of empirical attention has addressed the comorbidity of eating disorders and substance use disorders.

Comorbidity of Eating Disorders and Substance Use Disorders

Reviews of studies examining the comorbidity of eating disorders and substance use disorders have indicated that these disorders co-occur at high rates, particularly among individuals with bulimia nervosa or the binge eating/purging subtype of anorexia nervosa (Holderness, Brooks-Gunn, and Warren, 1994; Krahn, 1991; Lilenfeld, 2004; Mitchell, Pyle, Specker, and Hanson, 1992; Wolfe and Maisto, 2000). Although substance use disorders are not more common among obese binge eaters than controls (Telch and Stice, 1998; Yanovski, Nelson, Dubbert, and Spitzer, 1993), an uncontrolled, community-based study found similar rates of substance use disorders among women with bulimia nervosa and women with binge eating disorder who were unselected for weight status (Dohm et al., 2002). These latter findings suggest that substance misuse may be problematic among some women with binge eating disorder, perhaps particularly those who are not obese, although further controlled research is indicated. The converse effect has also been found: elevated rates of eating disorders and related symptoms have been consistently reported in substance misuse samples (e.g., Grilo et al., 1995; Holderness et al., 1994).

Sampling issues and Berkson's bias. The majority of the above comorbidity studies have been conducted with clinical samples, which result in artificially high rates of comorbidity because people with multiple disorders are more likely to pursue treatment—and thus be included in clinical samples—than those with only a single disorder (Berkson, 1946). Results from the majority of epidemiologic studies, which have the critical benefit of being comparatively unaffected by systematic recruitment biases, differ from clinical studies in suggesting that small but consistent associations exist between eating disorder symptoms and use and misuse of alcohol, tobacco, and illicit drugs (Bushnell et al., 1994; Garfinkel et al., 1995; Kendler et al., 1991; Schuckit et al., 1996; von Ranson, Iacono, and McGue, 2002; Welch and Fairburn, 1998). A minority of community-based studies have found no difference in rates of substance misuse among individuals with bulimia nervosa (Welch and Fairburn, 1996) and anorexia nervosa (Helzer and Pryzbeck, 1988) relative to community controls. Overall, the weight of the evidence indicates that eating disorders and substance misuse co-occur at somewhat higher than expected rates, but associations are not as strong as clinical studies initially demonstrated.

Specificity of comorbid associations. Rather than considering broad associations between these two classes of disorders, it may be important to consider the degree of specificity of association between eating disorders and substance misuse. In other words, is an eating disorder-substance misuse association largely limited to certain types of eating disorder symptoms—such as binge eating, purging, or both—or particular forms of substance misuse, such as nicotine, alcohol, or classes of illicit drugs? Identifying the breadth or specificity of associations between these types of problems has important implications for our understanding of the addiction model of eating disorders. As previously noted, comorbidity of substance misuse is believed to be largely limited to individuals with bulimic symptoms (e.g., Holderness et al., 1994; Lilenfeld, 2004). Some studies have found high rates of comorbidity of substance misuse—mostly alcohol dependence—among individuals with anorexia nervosa (Cantwell, Sturzenberger, Burroughs, Salkin, and Green, 1977; Henzel, 1984; Laessle, Kittl, Fichter, Wittchen, and Pirke, 1987; Schuckit et al., 1996) whereas others have not (Eckert,

Goldberg, Halmi, Casper, and Davis, 1982; Garfinkel, Moldofsky, and Garner, 1980). Unfortunately, because information on the subtype of anorexia nervosa was not included in these studies, it is impossible to determine the influence of recurrent binge eating or purging. Substances other than alcohol have been studied infrequently.

Are certain eating disorder symptoms differentially related to substance misuse? Few studies have systematically compared different subtypes of eating disorders—e.g., restricting anorexia nervosa, binge eating/purging anorexia, and bulimia nervosa—to ascertain whether prevalence rates are higher among eating disorders that involve binge eating, and fewer still have studied non-clinical samples. Consistent with the conclusion that strongest associations exist between bulimic symptoms and alcohol misuse, one large study of individuals recruited from clinical and other settings reported significantly higher rates of alcohol use disorders among women with anorexia nervosa and binge eating or bulimia nervosa, than among women with anorexia nervosa alone (Bulik et al., 2004). However, results from the only epidemiologic study that has examined comorbidity of substance misuse with different types of eating disorder symptoms are at odds with this finding. Specifically, this study found that restricting and bulimic symptoms were *both* modestly associated with adolescent girls' and women's use and misuse of nicotine, alcohol, and illicit drugs (von Ranson et al., 2002). Although some have argued that this study's results may be explained by elevated Type II error due to a lack of statistical power and use of conservative confidence intervals (Hudson, Hudson, and Pope, 2005), correlational analyses are presented that also tend to support the conclusion that no clear difference exists between restricting and bulimic symptoms and substance misuse (von Ranson et al., 2002). Specifically, similar levels of correlations were found between use and misuse of nicotine, alcohol, and illicit drugs across both bulimic and restricting disordered eating symptom groups in adolescent girls (range: $r = .05$ to .30). The strongest correlation ($r = .30$) occurred between nicotine use and binge eating and purging symptoms; the remaining correlations were all under $r = .20$. No clear pattern of associations of specific eating disorder symptoms with particular classes of substances emerged (von Ranson et al., 2002). Conclusions were limited by the fact that illicit drugs were grouped together in this study, rather than examined individually or separately by class, and no direct test was provided of correlation strength across types of eating disorder behavior.

In summary, existing evidence generally suggests that binge eating and purging behaviors are more strongly associated than restricting behaviors with substance misuse, particularly alcohol use disorders, although closer examination of associations among eating disorder symptoms and substance misuse among community samples is needed to clarify this issue more definitively. Future research should test associations of eating disorder symptoms with specific substances, including different types of illicit drugs. Individuals with eating disorders may have different motivations for using particular classes of drugs, including managing negative affect, avoiding problems, and appetite control (Stock, Goldberg, Corbett, and Katzman, 2002). It follows, then, that binge eating and purging may manifest different strengths and even directions of associations with varying substances. Individuals who are restricting their food intake may tend to avoid alcohol because of its caloric content, but may seek out illicit drugs that they believe may help them achieve their goal of weight loss. To our knowledge, no research has yet studied these questions.

Is comorbidity of eating disorders and substance misuse uniquely strong? The unique strength of the relationship between eating disorders and substance misuse, relative to other psychopathology commonly comorbid with eating disorders, is also at issue. Evidence of a uniquely strong relationship between two classes of problems would buttress claims that their association has specific etiologic importance.

Descriptive studies do not support the finding of a special, specific relationship between eating and substance use problems. In fact, some research indicates that rates of comorbidity of anxiety and mood disorders tend to exceed that of substance misuse among individuals with eating disorders or disordered eating attitudes and behaviors (Garfinkel et al., 1995; Laessle, Wittchen, Fichter, and Pirke, 1989; von Ranson, Iacono, and McGue, 2000, 2001). In contrast, other community-based research has described comparable odds of comorbidity of various mood, anxiety, and substance use disorders with eating disorders, with all odds ratios ranging from approximately 1.9 to 2.7, indicating that odds of having a comorbid disorder were two or more times higher among those with an eating disorders compared to those without (Wade, Bulik, Prescott, and Kendler, 2004). We are unaware of any studies that have provided direct, statistical comparisons of comorbidity rates of different psychiatric disorders with eating disorders to ascertain the relative strength of these relationships. Such research is needed to definitively answer the question of whether eating disorders and substance misuse share a uniquely strong relationship, although the weight of the current evidence suggests no such unique link exists.

Given the modest associations of substance use and misuse with eating disorder symptoms in nonclinical individuals, overall the empirical findings suggest that limited conclusions should be drawn about the importance of the comorbidity of eating and substance use problems. Nevertheless, an association appears to exist between these types of disorders.

Familial Transmission of Eating and Substance Use Disorders

Several studies have examined patterns of familial transmission of eating and substance use disorders for clues as to whether risk for one problem is associated with risk for the other across generations. Given the existing evidence that both eating disorders and substance misuse are substantially heritable (Bulik, Sullivan, Wade, and Kendler, 2000), a demonstration of shared risk for these problems would strongly suggest a common, possibly "addictive" etiology. However, research consistently indicates these disorders are not cross-transmitted in families (Kaye et al., 1996; Kendler et al., 1995; Schuckit et al., 1996), including when subsyndromal disordered eating-substance misuse associations within individuals are carefully separated from familial associations (von Ranson, McGue, and Iacono, 2003). Although as noted above, many believe that eating disorders and substance use disorders are the product of a common biological vulnerability (e.g., Jonas, 1990), the family study data clearly do not support this hypothesis.

Brain Circuits, Reward and Addiction

An intriguing area of research suggests there may be commonalities in neural circuitry in individuals with eating disorders and individuals with substance misuse. Specifically, addictive behaviors, such as those occurring in eating disorders, may stimulate the endogenous production of opiates, psycho-stimulants or other analogs of exogenous, addictive substances, as well as naturally occurring neurotransmitters (Grigson, 2002; Holden, 2001; Shaffer, 1996). Elevated levels of endogenous opioids have been reported in studies of anorexia nervosa, bulimia nervosa, and obesity (Grigson, 2002; Lesieur and Blume, 1993), and dopamine neurotransmission, which has been implicated in mediating reward and reinforcement systems in the brain, appears to play a role in eating behavior (Orford, 2001; Wang et al., 2001). Brain imaging research indicates that the availability of obese individuals' striatal dopamine D2 receptors is inversely proportional to their body mass index and is lower than in controls, and the lack of dopamine availability is hypothesized to impact motivation and reward circuit pathways in these individuals (Wang et al., 2001; Wang, Volkow, Thanos, and Fowler, 2004).

Although some addictions researchers believe that long-term changes in reward neural circuitry may help perpetuate behavioral addictions such as eating disorders (Holden, 2001), this theory remains largely speculative. Preliminary support exists for the theory that although bulimic behavior may be voluntary at first, over time it may become compulsive due to chronic dysregulation of brain and vagal nerve pathways (Faris et al., 2000; Holden, 2001). Data are correlational and the specificity of such changes in neural pathways to specific behaviors is unclear, but neurobiology is a promising area for future research.

EXERCISE ADDICTION

Some authors have argued that exercise may have addictive properties, including negative effects akin to dependence (Cockerill and Riddington, 1996). Many individuals with eating disorders, most commonly anorexia nervosa, exercise excessively, typically defined as exercising to the extent that it causes functional impairment or is maladaptive (Davis, Katzman, and Kirsh, 1999). Exercise dependence, then, is hypothesized to be a form of behavioral addiction that may be prominent in individuals with eating disorders. In a recent study that used criteria to define dependence on exercise that were adapted from a measure of severity of substance use disorders, almost half (48%) of a sample of 21 inpatients with anorexia nervosa met criteria for exercise dependence over the previous month (Klein et al., 2004). These authors also noted a strong, positive association of number of exercise dependence criteria met with a measure of anxiety disorder symptoms ($r = .76$), raising the possibility that anxiety may help cause or result from excessive exercise (Klein et al., 2004). These data support the view that many individuals with eating disorders exhibit symptoms of addiction to exercise behavior, and are consistent with other research supporting an association of compulsive exercise in girls with anorexia nervosa, obsessive-compulsive personality, and a propensity toward addiction (Davis et al., 1999). Future research is needed to examine cross-sectional and longitudinal associations among eating disorders, anxiety, and excessive exercise, particularly in nonclinical samples.

PERSONALITY TRAITS

Impulsiveness and negative emotionality. One potential explanation for the frequent co-occurrence of eating disorders and substance use disorders is that individuals with both disorders may manifest personality characteristics related to addiction-proneness (e.g., Feldman and Eysenck, 1986). Substance misuse and bulimic symptoms might both stem from a failure to control impulsive behavior, or failure to consider risks and consequences and a lack of deliberation (Lacey, 1993). Impulsiveness—also commonly termed impulsivity—is an important risk factor for and correlate of substance abuse. For example, evidence indicates that those who abuse substances are more impulsive than those who do not, high impulsivity in childhood predicts later development of substance abuse, and impulsivity negatively affects treatment (Moeller and Dougherty, 2002). The other broad personality dimension that has been associated with alcoholism is negative emotionality, or propensity to experience negative emotions such as anxiety or depression (Mulder, 2002). Negative emotionality and impulsivity may interact to increase risk for alcoholism. Results from a study of a large community sample of men and women indicated that those high in both negative emotionality and impulsivity had the highest rates of alcoholism (McGue, Slutske, Taylor, and Iacono, 1997).

Like substance misusers, individuals with bulimic behaviors and bulimia nervosa tend to be impulsive (e.g., Cassin and von Ranson, 2005; Fahy and Eisler, 1993; Feldman and Eysenck, 1986; Schmidt and Telch, 1990; Steiger, Puentes-Neuman, and Leung, 1991). In contrast, individuals with the restricting subtype of anorexia nervosa tend to be less impulsive than non-psychiatric controls (Fahy and Eisler, 1993). Impulsiveness in bulimia nervosa appears to extend beyond a general association of impulsiveness with psychopathology (Penas-Lledo, Vaz, Ramos, and Waller, 2002) and is associated with poorer outcome of bulimia nervosa treatment (Keel and Mitchell, 1997).

If behavioral symptoms of bulimia nervosa, namely binge eating and compensatory behaviors, are conceptualized as impulsive, might it follow that those with bulimia nervosa, because they manifest multiple "impulsive" symptoms (i.e., both binge eating and purging) tend to be more impulsive than binge eaters who do not routinely use compensatory behaviors? Put another way, is there evidence that bulimia nervosa involves more addictive behaviors than binge eating disorder? No data directly address this question, but two lines of evidence provide initial support for it. First, those with binge eating disorder tend to score intermediately between those with bulimia nervosa and those without eating disorders on measures of general and eating psychopathology (Fichter, Quadflieg, and Brandl, 1993; Hay and Fairburn, 1998; le Grange, Telch, and Agras, 1997) and most scales on a commonly used measure of personality psychopathology, the Minnesota Multiphasic Personality Inventory (Kirkley, Kolotkin, Hernandez, and Gallagher, 1992), as well as impulsivity (Schmidt and Telch, 1990). Second, binge eating severity and frequency are positively correlated with impulsivity in treatment-seeking women (de Zwaan et al., 1994). Collectively, these findings suggest that individuals with binge eating disorder may tend to fall between individuals with bulimia nervosa and non-eating disordered controls on indices of severity of impulsivity, among other psychological features.

An alternate view of the relationship of addiction-related personality traits to bulimic symptoms suggests that a subtype of people with bulimia nervosa have a propensity toward both impulsivity and negative emotionality. One study reported that women with bulimia nervosa and substance dependence tended to come from families that experienced problems with impulsivity and affective instability, suggesting that a familial vulnerability toward impulsivity and negative emotionality exists among those women who have both an eating disorder and substance dependence (Lilenfeld et al., 1997). According to this perspective, only those bulimic women with substance dependence should demonstrate substantially elevated impulsivity, whereas those women with bulimia but no comorbid substance dependence should be more behaviorally constrained.

On the other hand, some have suggested that, rather than reflecting a stable personality trait, impulsiveness may reflect erratic dietary patterns and emotional instability associated with bulimia nervosa. In particular, one study's findings showed that reductions in binge eating and purging were followed by decreases in emotional lability and other aspects of behavioral disinhibition (Ames-Frankel et al., 1992).

In sum, unravelling the degree to which impulsiveness is a cause of bulimic behaviors, an effect of bulimic behaviors, or both, requires further study. Longitudinal designs are needed to answer these questions. One approach would involve assessing impulsivity in individuals with bulimia nervosa before and after recovery, but the optimal, heavily resource-intensive approach would involve measuring impulsivity before and after the onset of eating disorder symptoms.

Sensitivity to reward. Another personality characteristic proposed as potentially important in the etiology of addiction is sensitivity to reward, or the propensity to derive pleasure or reward from reinforcers such as food or addictive drugs. Initial research supports a hypothesized association between sensitivity to reward and eating pathology. Sensitivity to reward was found to be positively associated with emotional overeating and body mass index in a recent study (Davis, Strachan, and Berkson, 2004). These authors theorized that this personality variable may place one at risk for overeating and overweight; however, longitudinal research is needed to test its validity. Relations among sensitivity to reward, negative emotionality, impulsivity, and eating disorders also remain to be explored.

Historical Variability in the Concept of Addiction

Any discussion of the validity of the addiction model of eating disorders should include consideration of the meaning of the term "addiction." Historically the limits of the concept of addiction have been inconsistently defined, yielding a moving target of sorts. The classical definition of addiction was quite broad, referring to a habitual or compulsive devotion to an object or activity (*Webster's II New Riverside University Dictionary*, 1988). Beginning in the late nineteenth century, the term "addiction" was increasingly narrowed, and restricted to situations where physical dependence on a chemical substance could be substantiated through the presence of tolerance or withdrawal symptomatology (Walters, 1999). "Addiction" became identified—overly so, in some critics' view—with psychoactive drugs that exert an effect on the central nervous system (Orford, 2001). More recently, the definition has reverted to its earlier status (American Psychiatric Association, 1994) and has been extended to substances that do not appear to promote physical dependence, as well as non-substance related activities (e.g., pathological gambling, sex addiction, work addiction, internet addiction) (Peele, 1977). According to this revised definition of addiction, any reinforcing behavior is potentially addictive (Walters and Gilbert, 2000).

An ongoing controversy regarding the boundaries of the concept of addiction has been reflected in the differing levels of inclusiveness of the definitions of addictive disorders included in various editions of the Diagnostic and Statistical Manual of Mental Disorders (DSM), the American Psychiatric Association's definitional bible. In DSM-III, the definition of substance use disorders was quite restrictive, requiring the presence of physiological dependence, evidenced by tolerance or withdrawal (American Psychiatric Association, 1980). Individuals' pattern of use was not sufficient by itself for the diagnosis of substance dependence. By contrast, the DSM-III-R class of "psychoactive substance use disorders" incorporated a much broader definition of substance dependence by eliminating the requirement that tolerance and withdrawal be present and by increasing the emphasis on aspects of compulsive use, including loss of control, taking more of the substance than was intended, continued use of a substance despite negative consequences, and the interference with social or occupational functioning (American Psychiatric Association, 1987; Miele, Tilly, First, and Frances, 1990). However, the diagnostic criteria explicitly referred to abuse and dependence of *psychoactive* substances to ensure that the diagnostic criteria were not misinterpreted to include non-psychoactive substances such as food (Rounsaville, Spitzer, and Williams, 1986). The DSM-IV substance use disorders work group considered returning to a somewhat narrower definition of dependence, requiring the presence of either tolerance or withdrawal in addition to the compulsive aspects or problematic consequences of substance use (Miele et al., 1990), but ended up retaining a broader definition which did not require the presence of either tolerance or withdrawal (American Psychiatric Association, 1994). Using this current, broader definition, a number of behavioral syndromes, particularly compulsive and impulsive disorders, appear similar to psychoactive substance dependence (American Psychiatric Association, 2000; Miele et al., 1990).

The Controversy Over Expanding the Concept of Addiction

Whether the concept of addiction should be expanded beyond substance abuse to include behavioral (i.e., non-psychoactive) addictions is quite controversial. Goodman (1990) notes that the DSM omits a number of behavioral syndromes characterized by a prominent addictive component, with the notable exception of pathological gambling. Orford (2001) advocates for broadening the concept of addiction to include not only excessive psychoactive substance use, but also excessive gambling, sexual activity, and eating. However, the DSM's recent return to a broad definition of addiction has been widely criticized both within and outside the mental health field. According to the revised classical definition of addiction, any reinforcing behavior is potentially addictive; thus, in theory, a person could can be addicted to virtually anything (Wilson, 1991). This definition has been roundly criticized because it is so vague, subjective, and all-inclusive that it is devoid of pragmatic value and may obscure important differences between addictions despite the similarities in overt presentation (Goodman, 1990; Miele et al., 1990; Walters and Gilbert, 2000). The broadening of the concept of addiction may also have the unintended effect of pathologizing normal behavior.

Kaminer (1990, p. 26) stated, "...what were once billed as bad habits and problems are now considered addictions."

It is important to consider the reasons why narrower or broader definitions of addiction are being advocated, as well as what practical consequences are anticipated by each of the proposed classifications (Marks, 1990a). Ultimately, the classification of behaviors as addictive may reflect the financial, social, and political concerns of clinicians and researchers (Marks, 1990b). As Jaffe noted, "the taxonomy we select depends on our objectives" (1990, p. 1425). There is no getting around the fact that determining the boundaries of addiction, as with defining other forms of psychopathology, is inherently subjective.

Clearly, issues of definition are fundamental in the debate over what constitutes an addiction. The concept of addiction is controversial in part because clinicians, researchers, social policy makers, and laypeople lack a common definition of addiction (Shaffer, 1996). For example, in one study, clients in a drug education class and addiction experts from the American Psychological Association were asked to define the concept of addiction (Walters and Gilbert, 2000). No single symptom or criterion was endorsed by more than half of either group (clients or experts), which highlights the nebulousness of this construct. Both clients and experts associated addiction with impaired control. Significant disagreement in how addiction was defined was found both between and within the client and expert groups. Experts tended to focus on the compulsive aspects of the behavior and the presence of physical dependence (i.e., tolerance and withdrawal), whereas clients emphasized needs and urges to continue a behavior. Clients provided broader definitions of addiction relative to experts and were more likely to include behavioral addictions. One possible impetus for some to desire a broader definition of addiction is that an addiction label may have a responsibility-easing effect, thus alleviating personal responsibility for undesirable behaviors (Walters and Gilbert, 2000).

In addition to the lack of agreement over the essential elements of addictive behavior, addiction is difficult to conceptualize because, like many forms of psychopathology, there are no definitive means (e.g., objective measures such as pharmacological tests) for determining whether a person has this problem. Instead, various indirect or suggestive indicators of addiction have been relied on, particularly the observable characteristics of tolerance and withdrawal (Peele, 1977). *Tolerance* is the need for increased doses of a substance to produce the desired effect and is inferred when an individual shows less of an effect from the taking of a substance over time. *Withdrawal* refers to the constellation of physiological symptoms (e.g., shivering, sweating, vomiting, fever, sleeplessness) that result from cessation of regular administration of the substance. Because the readily observable and quantifiable symptoms of tolerance and withdrawal are no longer required for a diagnosis of psychoactive substance dependence according to DSM, it has become more difficult to determine whether an individual suffers from an addiction (American Psychiatric Association, 1994). Before discussing whether complex problems such as eating disorders merit being considered addictions, it is necessary to come to some agreement about the meaning of addiction.

A Proposed Definition of Addiction

As noted earlier, substance dependence, as defined in the DSM (particularly DSM-III, which required the presence of tolerance and withdrawal), is commonly viewed as the prototypical addiction. Because "addiction" does not appear as a diagnosis or concept in existing diagnostic manuals, there is no gold standard definition by which to judge with any degree of certainty whether eating disorders are addictions (Shaffer, 1996). In contrast to substance dependence, people may be less inclined to classify compulsive eating or exercising as addictions because the behaviors are legal and generally more socially acceptable even when uncontrolled, and this acceptance may protect the individual from viewing himself or herself as an addict (Peele, 1977).

Whether eating disorders should be considered addictions hinges on the breadth of the definition of addiction selected. If we were to use an inclusive definition of addiction, such as one that describes behavioral addictions as maladaptive, repetitive sequences of behaviors (Bradley, 1990), many would agree that binge eating, gambling, and excessive attachment to one's work might all qualify as addictions. In contrast, many would agree that these behaviors would not qualify as addictions using a narrow definition that requires the ingestion of exogenous drugs, such as that proposed by Grinspoon and Bakalar (1976, p. 177): "Dependence is a state, psychic and sometimes also physical, resulting from the interaction between a living organism and a drug, characterized by behavioral and other responses that always include a compulsion to take the drug on a continuous or periodic basis in order to experience its psychic effects, and sometimes to avoid the discomfort of its absence." As noted earlier, some consider food to be a drug (Sheppard, 1993).

While these two definitions of addiction fall near the extremes of the spectrum, others fall closer to the centre. For example, Peele (1977, p. 103) proposes the following definition: "Addiction is any compulsive activity or involvement which decreases a person's ability to deal with other aspects of his life to the point where the activity or involvement comprises the dominant source of emotional reinforcement and identity for the person." Other proposed definitions of addiction that do not readily clarify whether eating disorders should be considered addictions include, "things or activities that can reliably and robustly shift subjective experience" (Shaffer, 1996, p. 464), "anything which is sufficiently compelling to engage a person's consciousness so that he can temporarily be relieved from awareness which he finds painful" (Peele, 1977, p. 120), and "a repetitive habit pattern that increases the risk of disease and/or associated personal and social problems" (Marlatt, Baer, Donovan, and Kivlahan, 1988, p. 224). Each definition raises issues depending on which elements are emphasized and how they are operationalized, or translated into concrete symptoms. No empirical data are available to inform the decision of which definition of addiction to adopt.

Goodman (1990) defines addiction as "a process whereby a behavior, that can function both to produce pleasure and to provide escape from internal discomfort, is employed in a pattern characterized by (1) recurrent failure to control the behavior (powerlessness) and (2) continuation of the behavior despite significant negative consequences (unmanageability)" (p. 1403). Recognizing the lack of a gold standard definition of addiction, Goodman (1990) was the first to propose a set of diagnostic criteria for what he termed "addictive disorder" by incorporating and adapting many of the criteria for DSM-III-R (American Psychiatric Association, 1987) psychoactive substance dependence (a chemical addiction) and pathological gambling (a behavioral or non-chemical addiction). Proposed diagnostic criteria for "addictive disorder" follow (Goodman, 1990, p. 1404):

a) Recurrent failure to resist impulses to engage in a specified behavior
b) Increasing sense of tension immediately prior to initiating the behavior
c) Pleasure or relief at the time of engaging in the behavior
d) A feeling of lack of control while engaging in the behavior
e) At least 5 of the following:
   1. Frequent preoccupation with the behavior or with activity that is preparatory to the behavior
   2. Frequent engaging in the behavior to a greater extent or over a longer period than intended
   3. Repeated efforts to reduce, control, or stop the behavior
   4. A great deal of time spent in activities necessary for the behavior, engaging in the behavior, or recovering from its effects
   5. Frequent engaging in the behavior when expected to fulfill occupational, academic, domestic, or social obligations
   6. Important social, occupational, or recreational activities given up or reduced because of the behavior
   7. Continuation of the behavior despite knowledge of having a persistent or recurrent social, financial, psychological, or physical problem that is caused or exacerbated by the behavior
   8. Tolerance: need to increase the intensity or frequency of the behavior in order to achieve the desired effect or diminished effect with continued behavior of the same intensity
   9. Restlessness or irritability if unable to engage in the behavior
f) Some symptoms of the disturbance have persisted for at least 1 month, or have occurred repeatedly over a longer period of time.

This proposed definition of addiction, which would subsume specific chemical and behavioral addictions, is less susceptible (though not immune) to criticism because it strikes a balance between being sufficiently broad to include some behavioral (non-chemical) addictions, but not overly encompassing so as to be devoid of pragmatic value. Note that it retains the concept of tolerance but omits that of withdrawal. Goodman (1990) notes that the criteria are actually more restrictive than those of the DSM disorders most commonly identified as addictive disorders (i.e., psychoactive substance dependence and pathological gambling) because the present definition requires that certain criteria be met for an individual to qualify for a diagnosis. In contrast, the "a la carte" approach to the definition of substance dependence in DSM-IV requires a minimum of three of seven criteria be met (American Psychiatric Association, 1994). Because Goodman's definition of addiction (1990) is both explicit and moderate in scope, we use his proposed criteria below to address the question of whether eating disorders should be considered addictions.

SIMILARITIES BETWEEN EATING DISORDERS AND ADDICTIONS

If tolerance and withdrawal are not regarded as essential, defining features of addictions, eating disorders may be considered to share salient features of substance dependence. Might eating disorders be a form of behavioral, non-chemical addiction? Note that exploring this possibility does not require the assumption that all individuals with an eating disorder would necessarily have an addiction. It is reasonable to assume that different developmental pathways may exist to an eating disorder, of which addiction to certain behaviors might be one. Moreover, defining an eating disorder as a form of addiction would depend on an individual's specific symptoms.

Proponents of an addiction model of eating disorders believe bulimia nervosa may be functionally interchangeable with other forms of addiction (e.g., Brisman and Siegel, 1984). Evidence suggests that addictions, including behavioral addictions, have reciprocity. That is, engaging in one form of addiction increases the risk for another, and addictions may covary: as one form decreases, another increases (Haylett, Stephenson, and Lefever, 2004). Empirical research addressing topics related to whether eating disorders are addictions has focused on the similarities of drug addiction with bulimic behavior (in the forms of bulimia nervosa, binge eating disorder, or anorexia nervosa, binge eating/purging type) to a much greater extent than with self-starvation (i.e., anorexia nervosa, restricting type), reflecting an emphasis on the symptom of loss of control of eating rather than on the compulsive dieting that occurs in restricting anorexia nervosa. A contrasting theory suggests that some individuals develop a dependence—or addiction—to starvation (Szmukler and Tantam, 1984). We are unaware of any published empirical research addressing this theory.

Some of the similarities between drug addiction and binge eating mentioned in the literature have included preoccupation with thoughts about the substance, craving for the substance, a repeated urge to use the substance, impairment of social and physical functioning, continued use of the substance despite adverse consequences, loss of control, repeated attempts to stop using the substance, mounting tension until the substance is used, guilt following use of the substance, gradual return of the urge and tension, and use of the substance to temporarily regulate emotions and relieve negative affect (Gold, Frost-Pineda, and Jacobs, 2003; Marks, 1990a; Walters, 1999; Wilson, 1991; Wilson, 2000). Interestingly, many of these symptoms are listed in Goodman's (1990) proposed diagnostic criteria for "addictive disorder"—specifically the four required symptoms (repeated urge to use the substance, mounting tension until the substance is used, use of the substance to temporarily regulate emotions and relieve negative affect, and loss of control while engaging in the behavior), as well as frequent preoccupation with and engagement in the behavior, repeated efforts to control or stop the behavior, and continuation of the behavior despite adverse consequences.

Binge eaters often report eating in response to emotional stress, such as tension, anxiety, anger, boredom, loneliness, or interpersonal conflict; binge eating is then often followed by additional negative affect or guilt, which leads to further binge eating (Abraham and Beumont, 1982; Lingswiler, Crowther, and Stephens, 1989). This self-reinforcing, cyclical pattern is similar to those seen in other states of psychological dependence or addiction (Weiner, 1998), as described in the hedonic homeostatic dysregulation theory of drug dependence maintenance (Koob and Le Moal, 2001). For example, the temporary decrease in anxiety and tension that accompanies both binge eating and self-induced vomiting has been likened to that associated with alcohol abuse (Cappell and Herman, 1972).

As previously discussed in detail, some have hypothesized that eating disorders and substance dependence may represent alternate manifestations of an inclination to engage in addictive behaviors (e.g., Yeary, 1987), possibly due to a shared genetic predisposition that might include common addictive personality characteristics (Bulik, 1987; Goodman, 1990; Holderness et al., 1994). Theorists have suggested that similar personality traits may be found in individuals with bulimia nervosa as those who abuse psychoactive substances, such as inability to regulate tension, the need for immediate gratification, poor impulse control, and fragile self-esteem (McDougall, 1989). Efforts to identify an "addictive personality" that describes individuals across a wide range of addictions, including both chemical and behavioral addictions, generally have not supported this hypothesis. Research has not identified a consistent personality profile for patients with eating disorders or alcohol dependence (Shaffer, 2000), which has led to skepticism about the existence of an underlying addictive personality that would define risk for one or both of these types of problems (Nathan, 1988; Wilson, 1991).

It is unclear, however, whether appropriately specific questions have not yet been asked. Perhaps a unidimensional "addictive personality" does not serve to convey risk for addictive behaviors. Instead, specific personality traits, or perhaps interactions between personality characteristics, may be important. For example, in one study patients with both anorexia nervosa and bulimia nervosa were found to have high scores on the Addiction Scale of the Eysenck Personality Questionnaire (Davis and Claridge, 1998). These authors suggested that high neuroticism (i.e., negative affect and emotional reactivity), which is characteristic of both anorexia nervosa and bulimia nervosa, is a fundamental feature of an addictive personality, and that secondary traits influence the form of the addiction—for example, high neuroticism combined with high introversion may predispose an individual to develop anorexia nervosa, whereas neuroticism combined with high psychoticism may predispose an individual to develop bulimia nervosa (Davis and Claridge, 1998). Although research has not supported a link with introversion or psychoticism and eating disorders, it has suggested that neuroticism combined with high persistence tend to be associated with anorexia nervosa, whereas neuroticism combined with novelty seeking/impulsivity tends to be associated with BN (Cassin and von Ranson, 2005).

Differences Between Eating Disorders and Addictions

Despite certain apparent similarities between eating disorders and substance dependence, there are important differences as well (Vandereycken, 1990). The features associated with physical dependence—tolerance and withdrawal—have rarely been described among patients with eating disorders (Vandereycken, 1990; Wilson, 1991; but see McAleavey and Fiumara, 2001). Thus, it is unlikely any individuals with eating disorders would endorse the symptom of tolerance found in Goodman's (1990) proposed criteria for "addictive disorder." Individuals with severe eating disorders often spend a great deal of time engaging in behaviors related to their eating disorder, recovering from its effects, or engaging in the behavior when expected to fulfill occupational, academic, domestic, or social obligations. It is clear that substantial social (Herzog, Keller, Lavori, and Ott, 1987; Mitchell, Hatsukami, Eckert, and Pyle, 1985), occupational (Mitchell, Soll, Eckert, Pyle, and Hatsukami, 1989), and functional (Mond et al., 2004; Newman et al., 1996) impairment occurs among individuals with symptoms and diagnoses of eating disorders. However, substantial individual differences in impairment exist, depending on the severity of the eating disorder (Herzog, Norman, Rigotti, and Pepose, 1986; Mond et al., 2004).

Addiction is unlikely to be an all-or-none phenomenon (Peele, 1977), and, as noted above, some individuals with binge eating disorder or bulimia nervosa may meet Goodman's (1990) criteria for "addictive disorder" whereas others may not. Relative to individuals who are dependent on psychoactive substances, some individuals with eating disorders may experience less interference with occupational, academic, recreational, social, and domestic activities, although, as noted above, it likely depends on the severity of the illness. No direct comparisons of level of impairment have been made. However, few people with addictions are impaired in every aspect of daily life (Shaffer, 1996), and certain addictions can be regulated without significant interference with one's health or daily functioning (Watson, 1999).

Distinctions Among Addiction, Dependence, Compulsion, and Impulsiveness

The term "compulsion," as in "compulsive overeating," has frequently been used synonymously with "addiction" and "dependence," yet there may be important differences among these terms. Behavioral addictions are often described as compulsive to denote an attempt to escape an aversive internal state (negative reinforcement), whereas dependence implies a strong attraction toward something, typically to achieve a pleasurable internal state (positive reinforcement) (Goodman, 1990; Marks, 1990a). Goodman (1990) suggests that addiction results from a combination of dependence and compulsion. As the definition of addiction has become more inclusive, boundaries among addictive, compulsive, and impulsive behaviors have become less clear (Miele et al., 1990). Impulsive and compulsive behaviors are distinguished on the basis of the underlying motivation that drives the behavior. Initially, similar to dependence, impulsive behavior aims to achieve some pleasure, whereas compulsive behavior aims to prevent subjective discomfort. However, as the impulsive behavior escalates in frequency it becomes less pleasurable and more compulsive in nature. Miele et al. (1990) note that many individuals with addictions are initially characterized by high impulsiveness, and then proceed to develop more compulsive characteristics (e.g., use of substance to evade dysphoric states).

According to one study's findings, the binge eating behavior of individuals with bulimia nervosa tended to be more compulsive in nature relative to those with binge eating disorder, whereas the eating behavior of those with binge eating disorder tended to be more impulsive in nature (Raymond et al., 1999); however, impulsive and compulsive characteristics were often present within the same individual. For example, Raymond et al. (1999) found the majority of individuals with bulimia nervosa and binge eating disorder reported a release of tension after binge eating (suggesting compulsive behavior); however, some also reported a sense of pleasure or gratification after binge eating (suggesting impulsive behavior).

Vandereycken (1990) argues that although the behavior of individuals with bulimia nervosa can be described as compulsive, it is the act of purging rather than binge eating that is compulsive, because purging is associated with greater anxiety reduction than binge eating.

ADDICTION MODELS OF EATING DISORDERS

As noted earlier, according to the addiction-as-disease model of eating disorders, binge eating results from a dependence on certain food substances, such as white flour and sugar, which certain individuals are powerless to control. It postulates that food addictions are formed early in childhood when refined carbohydrates are offered to susceptible children, triggering the addictive process (Sheppard, 1993). This addiction model proposes that certain genetically susceptible individuals are powerless over certain foods as a result of a "food allergy" or disease process, not a lack of willpower. The etiology of "food addiction" is thought to lie in a physiological, biochemical condition of the body that produces cravings for refined carbohydrates and other food substances (Sheppard, 1993). According to this approach, effective management of binge eating requires (1) an admission that one is powerless over food and (2) total abstinence from all offending or triggering foods (Bemis, 1985; Ronel and Libman, 2003; Stein, O'Byrne, Suminski, and Haddock, 1999). The self-help group Overeaters Anonymous (OA), modeled after Alcoholics Anonymous, is a direct outgrowth of the addiction-as-disease model approach toward eating disorder treatment. Another addictions-based self-help group, founded in 2000, is Eating Disorders Anonymous, which, in contrast to OA's admission of powerlessness over food, states "we are powerless over our eating disorder" (Eating Disorders Anonymous, 2005).

A more radical addiction model, the auto-addiction opioid model, posits that chronic eating disorders may be conceptualized as an addiction to the body's endogenous opioids, specifically the β-endorphins (Marrazzi and Luby, 1986). Appetite dysfunction (i.e., starvation and/or bingeing) and strenuous physical activity are both capable of stimulating endorphin activity. Because of their intrinsic reward properties, these endorphins may be as addictive as the exogenous opiates (Davis and Claridge, 1998). Huebner (1993) argues that anorexics differ from normal dieters in the way they are powerfully and addictively influenced by the endorphin changes induced by starvation and exercise, similar to the way drug addicts are powerfully and addictively influenced by exogenous substances. Although limited evidence addresses this theory, research suggests endogenous opioid peptides may mediate preference for palatable foods, especially those high in sugar and fat, perhaps particularly in women with bulimia nervosa (Drewnowski, Krahn, Demitrack, Nairn, and Gosnell, 1992, 1995).

Because binge eating appears to have both compulsive and impulsive components (Raymond et al., 1999), it has been suggested that optimal treatment should address both of these aspects. Psychotherapy and pharmacotherapy may help alleviate the internal discomforts from which the binge eating had provided escape, but it is equally important to foster the development of healthier, more adaptive resources for meeting the needs which the binge eating had served to gratify (Goodman, 1990). Supportive groups, including 12-step groups, may help achieve this goal (Goodman, 1990).

Overeaters Anonymous

The first OA meeting was held in the United States in January 1960 (Haddock and Dill, 1999). It was initially developed to provide support to compulsive overeaters, but was later expanded to include other eating problems, such as bulimia nervosa and anorexia nervosa (Suler and Bartholomew, 1986). Based on the addiction model, the OA philosophy states that food addiction and obesity are the result of a disease process rather than a lack of willpower or moral defect (Haddock and Dill, 1999). In order to arrest the disease process, the individual must rely on a higher power in order to control his or her food addiction. In 1990, an attempt was made to adapt the 12-step philosophy to the area of eating disorders, culminating in the publication of The Twelve Steps of Overeaters Anonymous (Johnson and Sansone, 1993).

The Twelve Steps of Overeaters Anonymous are:

1. We admitted we were powerless over food—that our lives had become unmanageable.
2. Came to believe that a Power greater than ourselves could restore us to sanity.
3. Made a decision to turn our will and our lives over to the care of God *as we understood Him*.
4. Made a searching and fearless moral inventory of ourselves.
5. Admitted to God, to ourselves, and to another human being the exact nature of our wrongs.
6. Were entirely ready to have God remove all these defects of character.
7. Humbly asked Him to remove our shortcomings.
8. Made a list of all persons we had harmed and became willing to make amends to them all.
9. Made direct amends to such people wherever possible, except when to do so would injure them or others.
10. Continued to take personal inventory and when we were wrong, promptly admitted it.
11. Sought through prayer and meditation to improve our conscious contact with God *as we understood Him*, praying only for knowledge of His will for us and the power to carry that out.
12. Having had a spiritual awakening as the result of these Steps, we tried to carry this message to compulsive overeaters and to practice these principles in all our affairs (Overeaters Anonymous, 2004).

Clinical anecdotes suggest that at times OA is "remarkably successful" when other treatments have failed, particularly with bulimia and compulsive overeating (McAleavey and Fiumara, 2001). Most members are reported to come to OA as a last resort following many unsuccessful attempts to control their eating, including drastic diets, psychological therapy, alternative therapies, or even surgery (Ronel and Libman, 2003). Unfortunately, the anonymous nature of OA makes difficult an empirical examination of the efficacy of participation.

A recent qualitative study described four major "transformations" experienced by members over the course of their involvement with OA: (1) enhancement of spirituality, (2) perception of the problem as a disease rather than lack of willpower, (3) acknowledgement of powerlessness and development of self-acceptance, and (4) formation of rewarding, supportive relations with others (Ronel and Libman, 2003). Although OA is not affiliated with any particular religious group and most members report that spirituality had not been an integral part of their lives prior to OA, the aspiration for spiritual growth is the basis for recovery. When OA members submit to a "Higher Power," they become aware of their powerlessness over the addiction disease process for which they are not held personally responsible. Conceptualizing binge eating as a disease beyond the individual's control diminishes feelings of failure and guilt which paradoxically enhances the importance of personal responsibility (Ronel and Libman, 2003). The establishment of group relationships further diminishes feelings of guilt and shame because group members share their experiences and feelings and receive support from one another. Furthermore, OA members learn to satisfy their psychological and emotional needs through relationships with others, rather than using food to deal with feelings of isolation and alienation (Ronel and Libman, 2003; Weiner, 1998).

Overeaters Anonymous has a number of additional benefits. OA simplifies very complex psychological processes and offers a very concrete plan of action which is easy for most members to understand (Johnson and Sansone, 1993). Self-help groups can also enhance self-efficacy and engender hope by helping members feel that they have achieved changes through their own efforts without the aid of a professional. In addition, OA is free, easy to join, and available at times when therapists may not be, e.g., late evenings and weekends (Weiner, 1998).

Criticisms of Addiction Models and Overeaters Anonymous

Although viewing food addiction as a disease may be helpful in alleviating individuals' sense of personal responsibility for binge eating and obesity, addiction models of eating disorders have been widely criticized on a number of grounds, summarized as follows. First, several key premises of the addiction model—e.g., the notions of food addiction and carbohydrate cravings—have received little empirical support (Stein et al., 1999). Second, the addiction model of eating disorders is overly simplistic. Third, the addiction model lacks parsimony in its explanation of eating disorder symptoms. Fourth, the addiction model does not distinguish between bulimia nervosa and binge eating disorder and does a poor job of accounting for anorexia nervosa. Fifth, treatments based on the addiction model (i.e., total abstinence from certain foods) are at odds with tenets of treatments for eating disorders that have demonstrated efficacy, such as cognitive-behavioral therapy. Each of these points is discussed in detail below.

Food Addiction

"Food addiction" is characterized by an obsession with food, chronic and compulsive binge eating despite adverse consequences, and loss of control over the amount of food eaten (Haddock and Dill, 1999). Although the addiction model and OA make reference to a food addiction, it is not the food itself, but an interaction between a person and food—in other words, the *relationship* of the addicted person with food—that defines addiction (Larkin and Griffiths, 1998; Shaffer, 1996). No evidence suggests that foods are inherently addictive, including refined carbohydrates. Most people incorrectly assume that addiction resides as a latent property of an object (e.g., "an addictive drug"; Shaffer, 1996). An individual may be addicted to a substance, but the substance itself is not addictive. Some take it a step further and argue that an addiction is an unnatural or acquired appetite. According to this perspective, food can never be addictive because it fills a basic need and is required for survival (Watson, 1999).

Carbohydrate Craving

There is no evidence to support the proposal that individuals with eating disorders experience food cravings as a direct consequence of consuming a "toxic" substance or "trigger" food to which they are sometimes said to be "allergic" (Bemis, 1985). Furthermore, there is no evidence that individuals with bulimia nervosa or binge eating disorder preferentially consume refined carbohydrates during a binge eating episode (Yanovski, 2003). The prevalence of carbohydrate cravings and rate of carbohydrate consumption do not differ significantly between nonobese individuals, obese binge eaters, and obese non-binge eaters (Drewnowski et al., 1992; Yanovski, 2003). The most salient difference between the binge episodes and non-binge meals of individuals with bulimia nervosa and binge eating disorder is the quantity of food consumed, not the proportion of carbohydrates (Walsh, Kissileff, Cassidy, and Dantzic, 1989; Yanovski et al., 1992). Research examining the effect of an opioid antagonist drug, naloxone, on the hedonic properties of sugar and fat found similar reductions in binge eaters and non-binge eaters but reduced the intake of sweet, high-fat foods only in binge eaters (Drewnowski et al., 1992, 1995).

Effects of Food on Mood

A critical assumption on which addiction models rest is that food has psychoactive, mood-altering properties (Haddock and Dill, 1999; Wilson, 1991). Well-controlled studies have provided little or no evidence to support this claim (see Haddock and Dill, 1999). The diets consumed by most individuals, including widely available foods, do not typically conform to the prerequisites for diets that alter neurotransmitter biosynthesis (Lieberman, Spring, and Garfield, 1986). In fact, foods demonstrate little pharmacological effect even when consumed in large quantities and in pure form (Lieberman et al., 1986). A review of studies examining the effects of carbohydrates on mood concluded that the mood-altering effects of carbohydrates are either subtle or nonexistent (Christensen, 1996), a fact which seriously challenges the validity of the addiction-as-disease model of eating disorders. Even if food was shown to regulate affect in some individuals, it would not necessarily follow that food is addictive because many activities regulate affect, including health-promoting activities such as meditation (Wilson, 2000).

Overly Simplistic

The addiction model has been criticized for being overly reductionistic (e.g., von Ranson et al., 2003). It focuses exclusively on binge eating because that behavior most closely resembles substance dependence, while neglecting other important characteristics of eating disorders such as purging, dietary restraint, and abnormal attitudes regarding weight and shape (Wilson, 1991; Wilson and Latner, 2001). Many clinicians have raised the objection that treatment programs based on the addiction model are superficial and do not address the deeper psychological issues of the patient, particularly commonly-comorbid personality disorders (Johnson and Sansone, 1993). The emphasis on abstinence from "toxic" foods is also problematic because, unlike drugs and alcohol, food has a role in healthy functioning and is essential for survival. Lifelong abstinence from particular foods is neither realistic nor desirable (Goodman, 1990; Wilson, 1991).

Lacks Parsimony

The biobehavioral explanations for food preoccupation and loss of control are somewhat convincing in the context of bulimia nervosa, but less so in the context of binge eating disorder and the restricting type of anorexia nervosa. Although individuals with binge eating disorder often attempt to abstain from certain "forbidden" foods, they are less inclined than those with bulimia nervosa to completely restrict their food intake so should be less susceptible to binge eating (Schmidt, 2000). Individuals with anorexia nervosa-restricting type significantly restrict their food intake, but do not engage in regular binge eating.

Binge eating may also result from the *abstinence violation effect* (Marlatt and Gordon, 1985), a phenomenon described in the addictions literature. According to this view as applied to eating disorders, individuals may categorize foods as either "safe" or "forbidden," and once a forbidden food has been consumed, they believe they have violated a dietary rule, give up, and binge eat. Of the foods consumed by bulimia nervosa patients during binge eating episodes, 69% contained individuals' forbidden foods (Kales, 1990). When forbidden foods are introduced back into the diet and normal, regular eating patterns are restored, both preoccupation and binge eating typically wane (Fairburn, Marcus, and Wilson, 1993).

Although certain similarities between eating disorders and substance dependence are noteworthy, we must also consider alternative explanations for addiction-like symptoms. Wilson (2000) contends that many of the symptoms (particularly preoccupation with food and loss of control) have biobehavioral explanations that do not invoke addiction, and notes that the most parsimonious explanation for these symptoms is that excessive dietary restriction and food deprivation trigger a specific constellation of physiological and psychological symptoms, including food preoccupation and binge eating. These symptoms can develop in food-deprived bulimics as they were shown to develop in healthy males participating in a longitudinal semi-starvation study (Keys, Brozek, Henschel, Mickelsen, and Taylor, 1950); thus, they should not be construed as withdrawal symptoms (Wilson and Latner, 2001). However, not all healthy, food-deprived males experienced food preoccupation and binge eating following food restriction, suggesting that there is not a direct, causal relationship between food deprivation and binge eating (Keys et al., 1950). Certain individuals may be genetically susceptible to developing binge eating symptoms.

Failure to Differentiate Among Eating Disorder Types

The addiction model has been criticized for failing to differentiate among the different eating disorders and obesity, treating them all as uniform addictive behavior. It is probably an overgeneralization to state that all eating disorders are addictions (McAleavey and Fiumara, 2001; Vandereycken, 1990). However, a lack of discrimination among eating disorder groups is expected because the addiction model conceptualizes eating disorders as one manifestation of a higher form of substance abuse (Wilson and Latner, 2001). However, there are important differences among the eating disorders. For example, unlike individuals with binge eating disorder, those with bulimia nervosa often restrict their food and compensate for their food consumption, yet, as noted above, the addiction model does not account for differences between those with bulimia nervosa and binge eating disorder. Individuals with the restricting type of anorexia nervosa restrict their food intake without regular bingeing or purging, suggesting they may be addicted to starvation, or the absence of food (Brumberg, 1988; Szmukler and Tantam, 1984). To complicate things even further, individuals with anorexia nervosa-binge/purge type restrict their food, binge, and purge, suggesting they are somehow simultaneously addicted both to food and to the absence of food. The addiction model does not adequately explain the paradox of a how a person can be addicted simultaneously to food and starvation (Wilson, 1991). The addiction model has difficulty accounting for the eating behavior of individual with anorexia nervosa since it does not closely resemble the unstructured and uncontrolled consumption of substance abusers (Wilson, 2000). To date no fine-grained analysis or explanation of different symptom patterns associated with eating disorders—such as presence or absence of binge eating, compensatory behavior, and food restriction—has been developed from an addiction-based perspective.

Lack of Empirical Evidence

Treatments based on the addiction model prescribe and promote dietary restraint, avoidance of certain foods, highly structured eating, and a sense of powerlessness (Bemis, 1985). In contrast, cognitive-behavioral therapy for bulimia nervosa encourages the establishment of regular, nutritionally balanced meals, the introduction of "forbidden" foods into a more flexible diet, and a reduction of abnormal attitudes about the importance of weight and shape. As stated above, the prescriptions of addictions-based treatments for eating disorders based on the addiction model (e.g., OA) have been widely criticized because they are at odds with empirically supported treatments for eating disorders and may actually contribute to their maintenance (Fairburn, 1997; Walsh, 1993). For example, abstinence rules promote dichotomous thinking (i.e., "safe" vs. "forbidden" foods) and may result in binge eating if a "forbidden" food is consumed due to the abstinence violation effect (Bemis, 1985). Conversely, abstinence rules may also serve as a form of "anorexic skills training" if an individual does abstain from all forbidden foods indefinitely (Vandereycken, 1990). Not only is there an absence of scientific evidence attesting to the value of the addictions model approach (Wilson, 1991; Wilson, 2000), but the therapeutic objectives of the addiction model may actually have unexpected, negative side effects (Parham, 1995). Vandereycken (1990) asserts that rather than abstaining from forbidden or toxic foods, the abstention target should be directed at all forms of abnormal weight reduction.

ADDITIONAL LIMITATIONS OF OVEREATERS ANONYMOUS

The efficacy of treatments based on the addiction model remain untested. Additionally, a number of additional, specific criticisms have been levied against the OA approach. First, because meetings are conducted by laypeople and run independently, there are no mechanisms for ensuring quality control across groups (Johnson and Sansone, 1993). Second, persuading group members that they are powerless to control their consumption of certain "toxic," addictive foods may promote feelings of low-self efficacy and pessimism regarding the likelihood of returning to a normal lifestyle (Haddock and Dill, 1999). Similarly, feminists assert that promoting powerlessness disempowers the largely female population of those with eating disorders, and also may backfire and intensify binge eating and/or prevent women from developing coping tools to actively deal with their problems (Ronel and Libman, 2003; van Wormer, 1994).

MAKING ADDICTIONS-BASED PSYCHOTHERAPIES MORE COMPATIBLE WITH EFFICACIOUS TREATMENTS FOR EATING DISORDERS

Although the addiction model and its treatment strategies suffer from a number of shortcomings, they may nonetheless contribute to the development of more comprehensive, effective approaches to the conceptualization and treatment of eating disorders (Goodman, 1990). As discussed earlier, OA has a number of beneficial aspects that group members find helpful, including a reliable social support system and alleviation of personal responsibility for binge eating. Criticisms of OA center on its three main themes: powerlessness, abstinence, and religious orientation. However, these aspects may be modified to make them more compatible with evidence-based treatments (Johnson and Sansone, 1993).

As suggested above, feminists have criticized the addiction model because the concept of powerlessness undermines the progress women have made toward greater empowerment, and eating disorders are theorized to stem in part from individuals' attempts to overcome feelings of powerlessness (Ronel and Libman, 2003; van Wormer, 1994). Thus, acknowledging powerlessness would be colluding with the primary problem of the patient. However, Johnson and Sansone (1993) note that the concept of powerlessness is more palatable when it is understood as an effort to identify those things that can be controlled versus those that cannot, rather than generalizing powerlessness to all aspects of life. Thus, OA members are not completely powerless over their problems, but rather, over some aspects of their eating behavior.

Clinicians who practice empirically supported treatments for eating disorders often disapprove of the notion of abstinence as applied to food. Food cannot be easily substituted for alcohol or drugs in the Twelve Steps because it cannot be eliminated from one's life as alcohol and drugs can. Furthermore, strict avoidance of certain foods can contribute to binge eating in some people (Keys et al., 1950). Cognitive-behavioral therapy encourages the development of a regular, flexible eating plan in which no foods are avoided. In a creative, constructive revision of OA's tenet regarding abstinence from carbohydrates, Johnson and Sansone (1993) recommend that rather than abstaining from specific foods, patients abstain from dieting, binge eating, purging, excessive exercise, and setting unrealistic weight expectations.

The religious orientation of 12-step programs makes some people uncomfortable and reluctant to participate in OA groups. However, OA does not insist people accept a specific definition of God and allows flexibility regarding who or what is chosen to define as their "higher power." It also makes a distinction between spirituality and religion. OA may appeal more broadly and be made compatible with more conventional forms of psychotherapy if the concept of higher power is interpreted in a spiritual rather than religious manner (Johnson and Sansone, 1993).

Although OA and other addictions-based approaches may be modified to be more compatible with evidence-based forms of psychotherapy, it does not necessarily follow that eating disorders should be treated using 12-step approaches even if they are conceptualized as addictions. Other psychotherapeutic options which have successfully been used to treat psychoactive substance use disorders include self-help manuals or guided self-help, motivational enhancement therapy, cognitive-behavioral therapy, behavioral self-control training, family therapy, relapse prevention, and medication (Hester and Miller, 1995). Behavioral self-control training and relapse prevention in particular are very similar to cognitive behavior therapy. Behavioral self-control training consists of behavioral techniques of goal setting, self-monitoring, managing consumption, rewarding goal attainment, functionally analyzing high-risk situations, and learning alternate coping skills (Hester and Miller, 1995). Relapse prevention aims to integrate behavioral skills training and cognitive intervention strategies to help individuals anticipate, identify, and manage high-risk situations to maintain behavioral change (Hester and Miller, 1995). Thus, even if a clinician conceptualizes eating disorders as forms of addiction, research evidence suggests that cognitive-behavioral therapy continues to be the optimal treatment for bulimia nervosa and binge eating disorder.

Conclusion

In this chapter, we have reviewed theory and evidence related to the view of eating disorders as addictions. In short, there is no simple answer to the question, "Are eating disorders addictions?" As discussed, the answer depends in part on our understanding of the terms we are using. First, how we define "addiction" is at issue, as there is no universally recognized definition for this crucial concept. Debate continues about the merits of considering behavioral addictions as equivalent to other, accepted forms of addiction, although recently there has been growing agreement among some experts that there may be benefits to broadening the view of addiction beyond the chemical addictions of alcohol and drug misuse (Holden, 2001). This broad conceptualization of addiction is consistent with definitions of substance use disorders found in the current edition of the DSM (American Psychiatric Association, 1994). However, whether eating disorders should be included among the problems defined as behavioral addictions also remains contested. Second, careful attention also needs to be paid to parsing the meaning of "eating disorders" in considering whether they constitute addictions. Do we mean binge eating, purging, other compensatory behaviors, food restriction, excessive exercise, associated cognitive symptoms, or some combination of the above? Systematic study of specific, carefully-defined eating disorder behaviors and subgroups is sorely needed to advance our understanding of whether eating disorders, or aspects of them, have addictive elements. Previous research has often made implicit assumptions about what element(s) of eating disorders may be addictive, yet little research has explicitly addressed the issue of specificity and no clear consensus has emerged.

Research is needed to shed light on the validity of the addiction model of eating disorders. Research on this topic is still at a nascent stage. Studies support neither the existence of a strong, overarching association of eating disorders with addictive disorders such as substance misuse nor the familial cross-transmission of these two types of problems. However, evidence exists for associations between the bulimic symptoms of binge eating and purging, on the one hand, and various indices of addiction, on the other. Promising areas of research examining possible links of eating disorders to addiction include the study of neural reward pathways and personality correlates and predictors of eating disorders. Surprisingly, no controlled studies have yet examined the efficacy of certain addictions-based approaches to treating eating disorders, despite their common use by community psychotherapists. As noted, a substantial minority of clinicians believe it is useful to conceptualize and treat eating disorder symptoms as addictive behaviors; the question remains if this belief is accurate or whether the perceived similarities between the two types of problems necessarily extend to the use of addiction-based treatments. It seems especially important to study the latter question because the tenets of 12-step-based treatments for eating disorders, in particular, run counter to those promoted by cognitive-behavior therapy, the evidence-based treatment of choice for bulimia nervosa and binge eating disorder.

At least two potential directions for future research related to addiction and eating disorders stand out. First, if addictive processes contribute to the development of eating pathology, then improved comprehension of these processes may help to refine prevention efforts directed at identifying those at risk and diminishing the numbers of people affected by eating disorders. Second, if addictive processes contribute to the maintenance of eating pathology, then understanding these processes better may yield new or improved treatment options. Conversely, if addictions-based treatments are found to be ineffective for eating disorders, the prompt dissemination of this information to therapists, patients, and others would be critical. These two important foci of knowledge acquisition related to the addiction model of eating disorders—etiology versus maintenance of eating pathology—should impact the direction of particular research questions.

For example, one means of gathering evidence addressing whether eating disorders should be considered addictions is through systematically researching how individuals with various eating disorders meet proposed criteria for addictive disorder (e.g., Goodman, 1990). According to Goodman's (1990) proposed diagnostic criteria, an undetermined subset of individuals with eating disorders would likely meet criteria for addictive disorder. Because

Goodman's (1990) proposed criteria refer to the existence of a behavior (e.g., eating), rather than the absence of a behavior (e.g., starving—the absence of normal eating patterns), it is unlikely anorexia nervosa-restricting type would be considered an addictive behavior (but see Szmukler and Tantam, 1984). Furthermore, the excessive exercise behaviors of half of a sample of inpatient women with anorexia nervosa was comparable to a series of adapted substance use disorder symptoms intended to assess addiction, although some substance use disorder criteria did not pertain to exercise (Klein et al., 2004). Of all the eating disordered behaviors, binge eating is most likely to be considered an addictive behavior, regardless of the formal diagnosis (i.e., anorexia nervosa-binge/purge type, bulimia nervosa-purging or non-purging type, binge eating disorder). Many individuals who binge eat report a recurrent failure to resist impulses to binge eat (criterion A), an increasing sense of tension immediately prior to initiating binge eating (criterion B), pleasure or relief at the time of binge eating (criterion C), and a feeling of lack of control while engaging in binge eating (criterion D). Many individuals who binge eat also report frequent preoccupation with binge eating (criterion E1), frequently engaging in binge eating (criterion E2), repeated efforts to reduce, control, or stop binge eating (criterion E3), and continuation of binge eating despite knowledge of adverse social, financial, psychological, or physical problems (criterion E7). Whether individuals who binge eat report spending a great deal of time binge eating or recovering from its effects (criterion E4), engaging in binge eating when expected to fulfill occupational, academic, domestic, or social obligations (criterion E5), or reducing their social, occupational, or recreational activities because of binge eating (criterion E6), likely depends on the severity of their binge eating disorder.

It is unlikely that many individuals who binge eat would endorse the symptom of tolerance (criterion E7). Although anecdotal evidence suggests that some individuals with eating disorders experience symptoms of physical dependence (i.e., requiring larger amounts of food to achieve the desired effect and experiencing headaches, sweats, irritability, mood swings, and panic when abstaining from certain foods; McAleavey and Fiumara, 2001), the empirical evidence is quite sparse (Wilson, 1991; Wilson, 2000) and it is uncertain whether these symptoms are truly indicative of tolerance and physical withdrawal. If binge eaters are addicted to food, their dependence on food appears to be a psychological one, without the presence of tolerance and physical withdrawal symptoms (Vandereycken, 1990).

In sum, whether individuals who binge eat would meet these or other criteria for addictive disorder would depend on the severity of their binge eating and the extent of its interference in their lives. To date, no empirical studies have been conducted to examine which particular diagnostic criteria individuals with anorexia nervosa, bulimia nervosa, and binge eating disorder would endorse, or what percentage of individuals with clinically significant eating disorders would meet full criteria for addictive disorder. Such research may help clarify the overlap between the concepts of addictive disorder and eating disorders, and so may ultimately help illuminate the etiology of eating disorders.

AUTHOR NOTE

The authors appreciate Kenneth Heng's assistance in compiling web-based data for this chapter.

REFERENCES

Abraham, S. F., and Beumont, P. J. (1982). How patients describe bulimia or binge eating. *Psychological Medicine, 12*(3), 625-635.

American Psychiatric Association. (1980). *Diagnostic and statistical manual of mental disorders* (3rd ed.). Washington, DC: Author.

American Psychiatric Association. (1987). *Diagnostic and statistical manual of mental disorders* (rev. 3rd ed.). Washington, DC: Author.

American Psychiatric Association. (1994). *Diagnostic and statistical manual of mental disorders* (4th ed.). Washington, DC: Author.

American Psychiatric Association. (2000). *Diagnostic and statistical manual of mental disorders* (4th edition, text revision ed.). Washington, DC: Author.

Ames-Frankel, J., Devlin, M. J., Walsh, B. T., Strasser, T. J., Sadik, C., Oldham, J. M., et al. (1992). Personality disorder diagnoses in patients with bulimia nervosa: Clinical correlates and changes with treatment. *Journal of Clinical Psychiatry, 53*(3), 90-96.

Bellodi, L., Cavallini, M. C., Bertelli, S., Chiapparino, D., Riboldi, C., and Smeraldi, E. (2001). Morbidity risk for obsessive-compulsive spectrum disorders in first-degree relatives of patients with eating disorders. *American Journal of Psychiatry, 158*(4), 563-569.

Bemis, K. M. (1985). "Abstinence" and "nonabstinence" models for the treatment of bulimia. *International Journal of Eating Disorders, 4*(4), 407-437.

Berkson, J. (1946). Limitations of the application of fourfold table analysis to hospital data. *Biometrics Bulletin, 1*, 47-53.

Bradley, B. P. (1990). Behavioural addictions: Common features and treatment implications. *British Journal of Addiction, 85*(11), 1417-1419.

Brisman, J., and Siegel, M. (1984). Bulimia and alcoholism: Two sides of the same coin? *Journal of Substance Abuse Treatment, 1*(2), 113-118.

Brumberg, J. J. (1988). *Fasting girls: The emergence of anorexia nervosa as a modern disease*. Cambridge, Mass.: Harvard University Press.

Bulik, C. M. (1987). Drug and alcohol abuse by bulimic women and their families. *American Journal of Psychiatry, 144*(12), 1604-1606.

Bulik, C. M., Klump, K. L., Thornton, L., Kaplan, A. S., Devlin, B., Fichter, M. M., et al. (2004). Alcohol use disorder comorbidity in eating disorders: A multicenter study. *Journal of Clinical Psychiatry, 65*(7), 1000-1006.

Bulik, C. M., Sullivan, P. F., Wade, T. D., and Kendler, K. S. (2000). Twin studies of eating disorders: A review. *International Journal of Eating Disorders, 27*(1), 2-20.

Bushnell, J. A., Wells, J. E., McKenzie, J. M., Hornblow, A. R., Oakley-Browne, M. A., and Joyce, P. R. (1994). Bulimia comorbidity in the general population and in the clinic. *Psychological Medicine, 24*(3), 605-611.

Cantwell, D. P., Sturzenberger, S., Burroughs, J., Salkin, B., and Green, J. K. (1977). Anorexia nervosa: An affective disorder? *Archives of General Psychiatry, 34*(9), 1087-1093.

Cappell, H., and Herman, C. P. (1972). Alcohol and tension reduction: A review. *Quarterly Journal of Studies on Alcohol, 33*(1-A), 33-64.

Cassin, S. E., and von Ranson, K. M. (2005). Personality and eating disorders: A decade in review. *Clinical Psychology Review, 25*, 895-916.

Christensen, L. (1996). *Diet-behavior relationships: Focus on depression*. Washington, DC: American Psychological Association.

Cockerill, I. M., and Riddington, M. E. (1996). Exercise dependence and associated disorders: A review. *Counselling Psychology Quarterly, 9*(2), 119-129.

Davis, C., and Claridge, G. (1998). The eating disorders as addiction: A psychobiological perspective. *Addictive Behaviors, 23*(4), 463-475.

Davis, C., Katzman, D. K., and Kirsh, C. (1999). Compulsive physical activity in adolescents with anorexia nervosa: A psychobehavioral spiral of pathology. *Journal of Nervous and Mental Disease, 187*(6), 336-342.

Davis, C., Strachan, S., and Berkson, M. (2004). Sensitivity to reward: Implications for overeating and overweight. *Appetite, 42*(2), 131-138.

de Zwaan, M., Mitchell, J. E., Seim, H. C., Specker, S. M., Pyle, R., Raymond, N., et al. (1994). Eating related and general psychopathology in obese females with binge eating disorder. *International Journal of Eating Disorders, 15*(1), 43-52.

Dohm, F. A., Striegel-Moore, R. H., Wilfley, D. E., Pike, K. M., Hook, J., and Fairburn, C. G. (2002). Self-harm and substance use in a community sample of Black and White women with binge eating disorder or bulimia nervosa. *International Journal of Eating Disorders, 32*(4), 389-400.

Drewnowski, A., Krahn, D. D., Demitrack, M. A., Nairn, K., and Gosnell, B. A. (1992). Taste responses and preferences for sweet high-fat foods: Evidence for opioid involvement. *Physiology and Behavior, 51*(2), 371-379.

Drewnowski, A., Krahn, D. D., Demitrack, M. A., Nairn, K., and Gosnell, B. A. (1995). Naloxone, an opiate blocker, reduces the consumption of sweet high-fat foods in obese and lean female binge eaters. *American Journal of Clinical Nutrition, 61*(6), 1206-1212.

Eating Disorders Anonymous. (2005). *The twelve steps*. Retrieved January 28, 2005, from *http://www.eatingdisordersanonymous.org/steps.html*

Eckert, E. D., Goldberg, S. C., Halmi, K. A., Casper, R. C., and Davis, J. M. (1982). Depression in anorexia nervosa. *Psychological Medicine, 12*(1), 115-122.

Fahy, T. A., and Eisler, I. (1993). Impulsivity and eating disorders. *British Journal of Psychiatry, 162*, 193-197.

Fairburn, C. G. (1997). Eating disorders. In D. M. Clark and C. G. Fairburn (Eds.), *Science and practice of cognitive behaviour therapy Oxford medical publications* (pp. 209-241). London: Oxford University Press.

Fairburn, C. G. (2002). Cognitive-behavioral therapy for bulimia nervosa. In C. G. Fairburn and K. D. Brownell (Eds.), *Eating disorders and obesity: A comprehensive handbook* (2nd ed.). New York: Guilford Press.

Fairburn, C. G., Marcus, M. D., and Wilson, G. T. (1993). Cognitive-behavioral therapy for binge eating and bulimia nervosa: A comprehensive treatment manual. In C. G. Fairburn and G. T. Wilson (Eds.), *Binge eating: Nature, assessment, and treatment* (pp. 361-404). New York, NY, USA: Guilford Press.

Faris, P. L., Kim, S. W., Meller, W. H., Goodale, R. L., Oakman, S. A., Hofbauer, R. D., et al. (2000). Effect of decreasing afferent vagal activity with ondansetron on symptoms of bulimia nervosa: A randomised, double-blind trial. *Lancet, 355*(9206), 792-797.

Feldman, J., and Eysenck, S. B. (1986). Addictive personality traits in bulimic patients. *Personality and Individual Differences, 7*(6), 923-926.

Fichter, M. M., Quadflieg, N., and Brandl, B. (1993). Recurrent overeating: An empirical comparison of binge eating disorder, bulimia nervosa, and obesity. *International Journal of Eating Disorders, 14*(1), 1-16.

Garfinkel, P. E., Lin, E., Goering, P., Spegg, C., Goldbloom, D. S., Kennedy, S., et al. (1995). Bulimia nervosa in a Canadian community sample: Prevalence and comparison of subgroups. *American Journal of Psychiatry, 152*(7), 1052-1058.

Garfinkel, P. E., Moldofsky, H., and Garner, D. M. (1980). The heterogeneity of anorexia nervosa: Bulimia as a distinct subgroup. *Archives of General Psychiatry, 37*(9), 1036-1040.

Gold, M. S., Frost-Pineda, K., and Jacobs, W. S. (2003). Overeating, binge eating, and eating disorders as addictions. *Psychiatric Annals, 33*(2), 117-122.

Goodman, A. (1990). Addiction: Definition and implications. *British Journal of Addiction, 85*(11), 1403-1408.

Grigson, P. S. (2002). Like drugs for chocolate: Separate rewards modulated by common mechanisms? *Physiology and Behavior, 76*(3), 389-395.

Grilo, C. M., Becker, D. F., Levy, K. N., Walker, M. L., Edell, W. S., and McGlashan, T. H. (1995). Eating disorders with and without substance use disorders: A comparative study of inpatients. *Comprehensive Psychiatry, 36*(4), 312-317.

Grinspoon, L., and Bakalar, J. (1976). *Cocaine: A drug and its social evolution*. New York: Basic Books.

Haddock, C. K., and Dill, P. L. (1999). The effects of food on mood and behavior: Implications for the addictions model of obesity and eating disorders. *Drugs and Society, 15*(1-2), 17-47.

Hay, P., and Fairburn, C. (1998). The validity of the DSM-IV scheme for classifying bulimic eating disorders. *International Journal of Eating Disorders, 23*(1), 7-15.

Haylett, S. A., Stephenson, G. M., and Lefever, R. M. H. (2004). Covariation in addictive behaviours: A study of addictive orientations using the Shorter PROMIS Questionnaire. *Addictive Behaviors, 29*(1), 61-71.

Helzer, J. E., and Pryzbeck, T. R. (1988). The co-occurrence of alcoholism with other psychiatric disorders in the general population and its impact on treatment. *Journal of Studies on Alcohol, 49*(3), 219-224.

Henzel, H. A. (1984). Diagnosing alcoholism in patients with anorexia nervosa. *American Journal of Drug and Alcohol Abuse, 10*(3), 461-466.

Herzog, D. B., Keller, M. B., Lavori, P. W., and Ott, I. L. (1987). Social impairment in bulimia. *International Journal of Eating Disorders, 6*(6), 741-747.

Herzog, D. B., Norman, D. K., Rigotti, N. A., and Pepose, M. (1986). Frequency of bulimic behaviors and associated social maladjustment in female graduate students. *Journal of Psychiatric Research, 20*(4), 355-361.

Hester, R. K., and Miller, W. R. (Eds.). (1995). *Handbook of alcoholism treatment approaches: Effective alternatives (2nd ed.)*. Needham Heights, MA: Allyn and Bacon.

Holden, C. (2001). "Behavioral" addictions: Do they exist? *Science, 294*(5544), 980-982.

Holderness, C. C., Brooks-Gunn, J., and Warren, M. P. (1994). Co-morbidity of eating disorders and substance abuse: Review of the literature. *International Journal of Eating Disorders, 16*(1), 1-34.

Hudson, J. I., Hudson, R. A., and Pope, H. G., Jr. (2005). Psychiatric comorbidity and eating disorders. In S. Wonderlich, J. E. Mitchell, M. de Zwaan and H. Steiger (Eds.), *Eating disorders review: Part I* (pp. 43-57). Oxford: Radcliffe Publishing.

Hudson, J. I., Mangweth, B., Pope, H. G., Jr., De Col, C., Hausmann, A., Gutweniger, S., et al. (2003). Family study of affective spectrum disorder. *Archives of General Psychiatry, 60*(2), 170-177.

Hudson, J. I., Pope, H. G., Jonas, J. M., and Yurgelun-Todd, D. (1983). Phenomenologic relationship of eating disorders to major affective disorder. *Psychiatry Research, 9*(4), 345-354.

Huebner, H. F. (1993). *Endorphins, eating disorders and other addictive behaviors.* New York, NY: W. W. Norton and Co, Inc.

Jaffe, J. H. (1990). Trivializing dependence. *British Journal of Addiction, 85*(11), 1425-1427.

Johnson, C. L., and Sansone, R. A. (1993). Integrating the twelve-step approach with traditional psychotherapy for the treatment of eating disorders. *International Journal of Eating Disorders, 14*(2), 121-134.

Johnson, C. L., and Taylor, C. (1996). Working with difficult-to-treat eating disorders using an integration of twelve-step and traditional psychotherapies. *Psychiatric Clinics of North America, 19*(4), 829-841.

Jonas, J. M. (1990). Do substance-abuse, including alcoholism, and bulimia covary? In L. D. Reid (Ed.), *Opioids, bulimia, and alcohol abuse and alcoholism* (pp. 247-258). New York: Springer-Verlag.

Kales, E. F. (1990). Macronutrient analysis of binge eating in bulimia. *Physiology and Behavior, 48*(6), 837-840.

Kaminer, W. (1990, February 11). Chances are you're codependent too. *New York Times Book Review,* pp. 26-27.

Kaye, W. H., Lilenfeld, L. R., Plotnicov, K., Merikangas, K. R., Nagy, L., Strober, M., et al. (1996). Bulimia nervosa and substance dependence: Association and family transmission. *Alcoholism: Clinical and Experimental Research, 20*(5), 878-881.

Keel, P. K., and Mitchell, J. E. (1997). Outcome in bulimia nervosa. *American Journal of Psychiatry, 154*(3), 313-321.

Kendler, K. S., MacLean, C., Neale, M., Kessler, R. C., Heath, A. C., and Eaves, L. J. (1991). The genetic epidemiology of bulimia nervosa. *American Journal of Psychiatry, 148*(12), 1627-1637.

Kendler, K. S., Walters, E. E., Neale, M. C., Kessler, R. C., Heath, A. C., and Eaves, L. J. (1995). The structure of the genetic and environmental risk factors for six major psychiatric disorders in women: Phobia, generalized anxiety disorder, panic disorder, bulimia, major depression, and alcoholism. *Archives of General Psychiatry, 52*(5), 374-383.

Keys, A., Brozek, J., Henschel, A., Mickelsen, O., and Taylor, H. L. (1950). *The biology of human starvation*. Minneapolis: University of Minnesota Press.

Kirkley, B. G., Kolotkin, R. L., Hernandez, J. T., and Gallagher, P. N. (1992). A comparison of binge-purgers, obese binge eaters, and obese nonbinge eaters on the MMPI. *International Journal of Eating Disorders, 12*(2), 221-228.

Klein, D. A., Bennett, A. S., Schebendach, J., Foltin, R. W., Devlin, M. J., and Walsh, B. T. (2004). Exercise "addiction" in anorexia nervosa: Model development and pilot data. *CNS Spectrums, 9*(7), 531-537.

Koob, G. F., and Le Moal, M. (2001). Drug addiction, dysregulation of reward, and allostasis. *Neuropsychopharmacology, 24*(2), 97-129.

Krahn, D. D. (1991). The relationship of eating disorders and substance abuse. *Journal of Substance Abuse, 3*(2), 239-253.

Lacey, J. H. (1993). Self-damaging and addictive behaviour in bulimia nervosa: A catchment area study. *British Journal of Psychiatry, 163*, 190-194.

Lacey, J. H., and Evans, C. D. (1986). The impulsivist: A multi-impulsive personality disorder. *British Journal of Addiction, 81*(5), 641-649.

Laessle, R. G., Kittl, S., Fichter, M. M., Wittchen, H.-U., and Pirke, K. M. (1987). Major affective disorder in anorexia nervosa and bulimia: A descriptive diagnostic study. *British Journal of Psychiatry, 151*, 785-789.

Laessle, R. G., Wittchen, H. U., Fichter, M. M., and Pirke, K.-M. (1989). The significance of subgroups of bulimia and anorexia nervosa: Lifetime frequency of psychiatric disorders. *International Journal of Eating Disorders, 8*(5), 569-574.

Larkin, M., and Griffiths, M. D. (1998). Response to Shaffer (1996): The case for a "complex systems" conceptualisation of addiction. *Journal of Gambling Studies, 14*(1), 73-82.

le Grange, D., Telch, C. F., and Agras, W. (1997). Eating and general psychopathology in a sample of Caucasian and ethnic minority subjects. *International Journal of Eating Disorders, 21*(3), 285-293.

Lesieur, H. R., and Blume, S. B. (1993). Pathological gambling, eating disorders, and the psychoactive substance use disorders. *Journal of Addictive Diseases, 12*(3), 89-102.

Lieberman, H. R., Spring, B. J., and Garfield, G. S. (1986). The behavioral effects of food constituents: strategies used in studies of amino acids, protein, carbohydrate and caffeine. *Nutrition Reviews, 44*, 61-70.

Lilenfeld, L. R., Kaye, W. H., Greeno, C. G., Merikangas, K. R., Plotnicov, K., Pollice, C., et al. (1997). Psychiatric disorders in women with bulimia nervosa and their first-degree relatives: Effects of comorbid substance dependence. *International Journal of Eating Disorders, 22*(3), 253-264.

Lilenfeld, L. R., Kaye, W. H., Greeno, C. G., Merikangas, K. R., Plotnicov, K., Pollice, C., et al. (1998). A controlled family study of anorexia nervosa and bulimia nervosa: Psychiatric disorders in first-degree relatives and effects of proband comorbidity. *Archives of General Psychiatry, 55*(7), 603-610.

Lilenfeld, L. R. R. (2004). Psychiatric comorbidity associated with anorexia nervosa, bulimia nervosa, and binge eating disorder. In T. D. Brewerton (Ed.), *Clinical handbook of eating disorders: An integrated approach* (pp. 183-207). New York: Marcel Dekker.

Lingswiler, V. M., Crowther, J. H., and Stephens, M. A. (1989). Affective and cognitive antecedents to eating episodes in bulimia and binge eating. *International Journal of Eating Disorders, 8*(5), 533-539.

Marks, I. (1990a). Behavioural (non-chemical) addictions. *British Journal of Addiction, 85*(11), 1389-1394.

Marks, I. (1990b). Reply to comments on "Behavioural (non-chemical) addictions." *British Journal of Addiction, 85*(11), 1429-1431.

Marlatt, G., Baer, J. S., Donovan, D. M., and Kivlahan, D. R. (1988). Addictive behaviors: Etiology and treatment. *Annual Review of Psychology, 39*, 223-252.

Marlatt, G. A., and Gordon, J. R. (Eds.). (1985). *Relapse prevention: Maintenance strategies in the treatment of addictive behaviors*. New York: Guilford Press.

Marrazzi, M. A., and Luby, E. D. (1986). An auto-addiction opioid model of chronic anorexia nervosa. *International Journal of Eating Disorders, 5*(2), 191-208.

McAleavey, K. M. A., and Fiumara, M. C. (2001). Eating disorders: Are they addictions? A dialogue. *Journal of Social Work Practice in the Addictions, 1*(2), 107-113.

McDougall, J. (1989). *Theaters of the body: A psychoanalytic approach to psychosomatic illness.* New York, NY: W. W. Norton and Co, Inc.

McGue, M., Slutske, W., Taylor, J., and Iacono, W. G. (1997). Personality and substance use disorders: I. Effects of gender and alcoholism subtype. *Alcoholism: Clinical and Experimental Research, 21*(3), 513-520.

Miele, G. M., Tilly, S. M., First, M., and Frances, A. (1990). The definition of dependence and behavioural addictions. *British Journal of Addiction, 85*(11), 1421-1423.

Mitchell, J. E., Hatsukami, D., Eckert, E. D., and Pyle, R. L. (1985). Characteristics of 275 patients with bulimia. *American Journal of Psychiatry, 142*(4), 482-485.

Mitchell, J. E., Pyle, R. L., Specker, S., and Hanson, K. (1992). Eating disorders and chemical dependency. In J. Yager, H. E. Gwirtsman and C. K. Edelstein (Eds.), *Special problems in managing eating disorders* (pp. 1-14). Washington, DC: American Psychiatric Press.

Mitchell, J. E., Soll, E., Eckert, E. O., Pyle, R. L., and Hatsukami, D. (1989). The changing population of bulimia nervosa patients in an eating disorders program. *Hospital and Community Psychiatry, 40*(11), 1188-1189.

Moeller, F., and Dougherty, D. M. (2002). Impulsivity and substance abuse: What is the connection? *Addictive Disorders and Their Treatment, 1*(1), 3-10.

Mond, J., Rodgers, B., Hay, P., Korten, A., Owen, C., and Beumont, P. (2004). Disability associated with community cases of commonly occuring eating disorders. *Australian and New Zealand Journal of Public Health, 28*(3), 246-251.

Mulder, R. T. (2002). Alcoholism and personality. *Australian and New Zealand Journal of Psychiatry, 36*(1), 44-51.

Nathan, P. E. (1988). The addictive personality is the behavior of the addict. *Journal of Consulting and Clinical Psychology, 56*(2), 183-188.

Newman, D. L., Moffitt, T. E., Caspi, A., Magdol, L., Silva, P. A., and Stanton, W. R. (1996). Psychiatric disorder in a birth cohort of young adults: Prevalence, comorbidity, clinical significance, and new case incidence from ages 11-21. *Journal of Consulting and Clinical Psychology, 64*(3), 552-562.

Orford, J. (2001). Addiction as excessive appetite. *Addiction, 96*(1), 15-31.

Overeaters Anonymous. (2004). *Twelve steps.* Retrieved July 28, 2004, from *www.overeatersanonymous.org/twelve_steps.html*

Parham, E. S. (1995). Compulsive eating: Applying a medical addiction model. In T. B. Van Itallie and A. P. Simopoulos (Eds.), *Obesity: New directions in assessment and management.* Philadelphia, PA: Charles Press.

Peele, S. (1977). Redefining addiction. I. Making addiction a scientifically and socially useful concept. *International Journal of Health Services, 7*(1), 103-124.

Penas-Lledo, E., Vaz, F. J., Ramos, M., and Waller, G. (2002). Impulsive behaviors in bulimic patients: Relation to general psychopathology. *International Journal of Eating Disorders, 32*(1), 98-102.

Raymond, N. C., Neumeyer, B., Thuras, P., Weller, C. L., Eckert, E. D., Crow, S. J., et al. (1999). Compulsive and impulsive traits in individuals with obese binge eating disorder and bulimia nervosa. *Eating Disorders: The Journal of Treatment and Prevention, 7*(4), 299-317.

Reid, M., and Burr, J. (2000). Are eating disorders feminine addictions? *Addiction Research, 8*(3), 203-210.

Riley, E. A. (1991). Eating disorders as addictive behavior: Integrating 12-step programs into treatment planning. *Nursing Clinics of North America, 26*(3), 715-726.

Ronel, N., and Libman, G. (2003). Eating disorders and recovery: Lessons from Overeaters Anonymous. *Clinical Social Work Journal, 31*(2), 155-177.

Rounsaville, B. J., Spitzer, R. L., and Williams, J. B. (1986). Proposed changes in DSM-III substance use disorders: Description and rationale. *American Journal of Psychiatry, 143*(4), 463-468.

Schmidt, N. B., and Telch, M. J. (1990). Prevalence of personality disorders among bulimics, nonbulimic binge eaters, and normal controls. *Journal of Psychopathology and Behavioral Assessment, 12*(2), 169-185.

Schmidt, U. (2000). Binge eating and binge eating disorder. *European Eating Disorders Review, 8*(5), 340-343.

Schuckit, M. A., Tipp, J. E., Anthenelli, R. M., Bucholz, K. K., Hesselbrock, V. M., and Nurnberger, J. I. J. (1996). Anorexia nervosa and bulimia nervosa in alcohol-dependent men and women and their relatives. *American Journal of Psychiatry, 153*(1), 74-82.

Shaffer, H. J. (1996). Understanding the means and objects of addiction: Technology, the Internet and gambling. *Journal of Gambling Studies, 12*(4), 461-469.

Shaffer, H. J. (2000). Addictive personality. In A. E. Kazdin (Ed.), *Encyclopedia of psychology* (Vol. 1, pp. 35-36). Washington DC, US: American Psychological Association.

Sheppard, K. (1993). *Food addiction: The body knows.* Deerfield Beach, FL: Health Communications, Inc.

Steiger, H., Puentes-Neuman, G., and Leung, F. Y. K. (1991). Personality and family features of adolescent girls with eating symptoms: Evidence for restricter/binger differences in a nonclinical population. *Addictive Behaviors, 16*(5), 303-314.

Stein, R. J., O'Byrne, K. K., Suminski, R. R., and Haddock, C. K. (1999). Etiology and treatment of obesity in adults and children: Implications for the addiction model. *Drugs and Society, 15*(1-2), 103-121.

Stock, S. L., Goldberg, E., Corbett, S., and Katzman, D. K. (2002). Substance use in female adolescents with eating disorders. *Journal of Adolescent Health, 31*(2), 176-182.

Suler, J., and Bartholomew, E. (1986). The ideology of Overeaters Anonymous. *Social Policy, 16*(4), 48-53.

Szmukler, G. I., and Tantam, D. (1984). Anorexia nervosa: Starvation dependence. *British Journal of Medical Psychology, 57*(Pt 4), 303-310.

Telch, C. F., and Stice, E. (1998). Psychiatric comorbidity in women with binge eating disorder: Prevalence rates from a non-treatment-seeking sample. *Journal of Consulting and Clinical Psychology, 66*(5), 768-776.

Thompson-Brenner, H., Glass, S., and Westen, D. (2003). A multidimensional meta-analysis of psychotherapy for bulimia nervosa. *Clinical Psychology-Science and Practice, 10*(3), 269-287.

Trotzky, A. S. (2002). The treatment of eating disorders as addiction among adolescent females. *International Journal of Adolescent Medicine and Health, 14*(2), 269-274.

van Wormer, K. (1994). "Hi, I'm Jane; I'm a compulsive overeater". In P. Fallon, M. A. Katzman and S. C. Wooley (Eds.), *Feminist perspectives on eating disorders* (pp. 287-298). New York: The Guilford Press.

Vandereycken, W. (1990). The addiction model in eating disorders: Some critical remarks and a selected bibliography. *International Journal of Eating Disorders, 9*(1), 95-101.

von Ranson, K. M., Iacono, W. G., and McGue, M. (2002). Disordered eating and substance use in an epidemiological sample: I. Associations within individuals. *International Journal of Eating Disorders, 31*(4), 389-403.

von Ranson, K. M., Iacono, W. G., and McGue, M. K. (2000, November). *Are disordered eating and substance abuse uniquely associated? Psychiatric comorbidity and disordered eating in adolescent girls.* Paper presented at the Eating Disorders Research Society annual meeting, Prien, Germany.

von Ranson, K. M., Iacono, W. G., and McGue, M. K. (2001, November). *Are disordered eating and substance abuse uniquely associated in women?* Paper presented at the Eating Disorders Research Society annual meeting, Bernalillo, New Mexico.

von Ranson, K. M., McGue, M., and Iacono, W. G. (2003). Disordered eating and substance use in an epidemiological sample: II. Associations within families. *Psychology of Addictive Behaviors, 17*(3), 193-202.

von Ranson, K. M., and Robinson, K. E. (2006). Who is providing what type of psychotherapy to eating disorder clients?: A survey. *International Journal of Eating Disorders,39*(1), 27-34.

Wade, T. D., Bulik, C. M., Prescott, C. A., and Kendler, K. S. (2004). Sex influences on shared risk factors for bulimia nervosa and other psychiatric disorders. *Archives of General Psychiatry, 61*(3), 251-256.

Walsh, B. (1993). Binge eating in bulimia nervosa. In C. G. Fairburn and G. Wilson (Eds.), *Binge eating: Nature, assessment, and treatment* (pp. 37-49). New York, NY: Guilford Press.

Walsh, B. T., Kissileff, H. R., Cassidy, S. M., and Dantzic, S. (1989). Eating behavior of women with bulimia. *Archives of General Psychiatry, 46*(1), 54-58.

Walters, G. D. (1999). *The addiction concept: Working hypothesis or self-fulfilling prophesy?* Needham Heights, MA: Allyn and Bacon.

Walters, G. D., and Gilbert, A. A. (2000). Defining addiction: Contrasting views of clients and experts. *Addiction Research, 8*(3), 211-220.

Wang, G. J., Volkow, N. D., Logan, J., Pappas, N. R., Wong, C. T., Zhu, W., et al. (2001). Brain dopamine and obesity. *Lancet, 357*(9253), 354-357.

Wang, G. J., Volkow, N. D., Thanos, P. K., and Fowler, J. S. (2004). Similarity between obesity and drug addiction as assessed by neurofunctional imaging: A concept review. *Journal of Addictive Diseases, 23*(3), 39-53.

Watson, G. (1999). Disordered appetites: Addiction, compulsion, and dependence. In J. Elster (Ed.), *Addiction: Entries and exits* (pp. 3-28). New York, NY: Russell Sage Foundation.

Webster's II New Riverside University Dictionary. (1988). Boston, MA: Houghton Mifflin.

Weiner, S. (1998). The addiction of overeating: Self-help groups as treatment models. *Journal of Clinical Psychology, 54*(2), 163-167.

Welch, S. L., and Fairburn, C. G. (1996). Impulsivity or comorbidity in bulimia nervosa: A controlled study of deliberate self-harm and alcohol and drug misuse in a community sample. *British Journal of Psychiatry, 169*(4), 451-458.

Welch, S. L., and Fairburn, C. G. (1998). Smoking and bulimia nervosa. *International Journal of Eating Disorders, 23*(4), 433-437.

Wilson, G. T. (1991). The addiction model of eating disorders: A critical analysis. *Advances in Behaviour Research and Therapy, 13*(1), 27-72.

Wilson, G. T. (1993). Binge eating and addictive disorders. In C. G. Fairburn and G. T. Wilson (Eds.), *Binge eating: Nature, assessment, and treatment* (pp. 97-120). New York: Guilford Press.

Wilson, G. T. (1999). Eating disorders and addiction. *Drugs and Society, 15*(1-2), 87-101.

Wilson, G. T. (2000). Eating disorders and addiction. In W. S. C. Poston and C. K. Haddock (Eds.), *Food as a drug* (pp. 87-101). Binghamton, NY: Haworth Press.

Wilson, G. T. (2002). Eating disorders and addictive disorders. In C. G. Fairburn and K. D. Brownell (Eds.), *Eating disorders and obesity: A comprehensive handbook* (2nd ed., pp. 199-203). New York: Guilford Press.

Wilson, G. T., and Latner, J. D. (2001). Eating disorders and addiction. In M. M. Hetherington (Ed.), *Food cravings and addiction* (1 ed., pp. 585-605). London: Leatherhead Publishing.

Wilson, G. T., and Pike, K. M. (2001). Eating disorders. In D. H. Barlow (Ed.), *Clinical handbook of psychological disorders* (3rd ed., pp. 332-375). New York: Guilford Press.

Wolfe, W. L., and Maisto, S. A. (2000). The relationship between eating disorders and substance use: Moving beyond co-prevalence research. *Clinical Psychology Review, 20*(5), 617-631.

Yanovski, S. (2003). Sugar and fat: cravings and aversions. *Journal of Nutrition, 133*(3), 835S-837S.

Yanovski, S. Z., Leet, M., Yanovski, J. A., Flood, M., Gold, P. W., Kissileff, H. R., et al. (1992). Food selection and intake of obese women with binge-eating disorder. *American Journal of Clinical Nutrition, 56*(6), 975-980.

Yanovski, S. Z., Nelson, J. E., Dubbert, B. K., and Spitzer, R. L. (1993). Association of binge eating disorder and psychiatric comorbidity in obese subjects. *American Journal of Psychiatry, 150*(10), 1472-1479.

Yeary, J. (1987). The use of Overeaters Anonymous in the treatment of eating disorders. *Journal of Psychoactive Drugs, 19*(3), 303-309.

In: Eating Disorders and Weight Loss Research
Editor: Jerome S. Rubin, pp. 39-65
ISBN 1-60021-334-0

Chapter 2

GENDER-RELATED ASPECTS OF EATING DISORDERS: A PSYCHOSOCIAL VIEW

Rosa Behar [1]
Department of Psychiatry, University of Valparaiso,
Mailbox 92-V, Valparaiso, Chile

PRELIMINARY CONSIDERATIONS

Various biological, psychological, and sociocultural factors have been considered in the attempt to understand the etiology of eating pathologies such as anorexia nervosa and bulimia nervosa. Psychosexual issues are neither sufficient nor necessary for the development of an eating disorder in a young person, and it should be considered as only one factor in the multidimensional, multifactorial framework needed to clarify this complex and still poorly understood set of disorders (Fornari and Dancyger, 2003).

In particular, gender roles and sociocultural expectations appear strongly implicated in the development of eating disorders, since anorexia nervosa and bulimia nervosa occur predominantly among women (Garfinfel and Garner 1982; Hsu 1990). This is frequently attributed to the continued emphasis on physical attractiveness and a thin physique for women (Polivy *et al*, 1986). In consequence, women reportedly express greater dissatisfaction about their bodies (Fallon and Rozin 1985), more concern with appearance and body weight (Pliner *et al*, 1990), and more frequently engage in weight-control efforts (Herman and Polivy 1980; Polivy and Herman 1983).

Since at least 90 per cent of eating disordered patients are females, then it would therefore seem plausible to suggest that the female role might play a part in the genesis of these pathologies. This fact strongly supports that the meaning of femininity in Western society has some relationship with the development of eating problems (Garfinkel and Garner, 1982; Garner *et al*, 1983; Garner *et al*, 1985).

Eating disorders are common, serious illnesses that present major challenges to physicians and other health care professionals. Sociocultural body norms for ideal size and

[1] Professor of the Department of Psychiatry, University of Valparaiso, Mailbox 92-V, Valparaiso, CHILE

shape may be reinforced by participation in activities, sports, or membership in groups that promotes weight loss and shape change. Eating disorders are furthermore reinforced when high status individuals (e.g. parents, teachers, coaches, doctors) encourage a susceptible individual to diet. Studies indicate that a complex combination of genetic and sociocultural-developmental factors is responsible for the onset of these illnesses (Andersen, 1999).

Society and Eating Disorders

Eating disorders can also be regarded as a cultural phenomenon and a social problem, and may illuminate the influence of culture on psychopathology better than other disorders. Nevertheless, the role of sociocultural factors continues to be underemphasized in the theoretical and empirical literature and the meaning of sociocultural influences needs to be closely examined.

Culture has been identified as one of the etiological factors leading to the development of these syndromes. Rates of these pathologies appear to vary among different cultures and to change across time as cultures evolve. Additionally, eating disorders appear to be more widespread among contemporary cultural groups than was previously believed. It seems likely that the sociocultural factors that have occurred across time and throughout different contemporary societies play a role in the emergence of these disorders. In many non Western societies, plumpness is considered attractive and desirable, and may be associated with prosperity, fertility, success and economic security (Nassar, 1988). In such cultures, eating disorders are found much less commonly than in Western nations. Anorexia nervosa has been described as a possible "culture-bound syndrome", with roots in Western cultural values and conflicts (Prince, 1983).

Cultures in which female social roles are restricted appear to have lower rates of eating disorders, reminiscent of the lower rates observed during historical eras in which women lacked choices. For example, some modern affluent Muslim societies limit the social behavior of women according to male dictates; in such societies, eating disorders are virtually unknown. This supports the notion that freedom for women, as well as affluence, are sociocultural factors that may predispose to the development of eating disorders (Bemporad, 1997).

Eating disorders may, in fact, be more prevalent within various cultural groups than previously recognized, as Western values are becoming more widely accepted. Historical and cross-cultural experiences suggest that cultural change, itself, may be associated with increased vulnerability to eating disorders, especially when values about physical aesthetics are involved. Such change may occur across time within a given society, or on an individual level, as when an immigrant moves into a new culture. In addition, cultural factors such as affluence and freedom of choice for women may play a role in the development of these pathologies (Bemporad, 1997; Miller and Pumariega, 2001).

Contrary to the biological determinism perspective, the sociocultural view of gender roles states that gender roles and stereotypes develop within a culture and are then perpetuated by that culture. Individuals within the culture are expected to conform to these norms, and are socialized in manners which constantly reinforce the beliefs and behaviors which are prescribed and presupposed for them.

The biological view of gender roles states that the differentiated gender roles which exist in our society are the products of our evolution, and are inextricably linked with abilities predominant in one gender or the other which are biologically determined. The roles prescribed for each sex are based on physical abilities and properties of that sex, such as intelligence, brain lateralization, and differing hormone levels. Implicit within this view is the belief that these roles are both desirable and immutable (Singleton, 1987).

The assumption that sex roles are biological, and therefore unchanging, can be refuted by the simple observable fact that sex roles, even within our society, have changed and are in the process of changing. Thus far, the focus of gender eating-disorders research has been on gender role adoption. However, being female means more than adopting a particular gender role. It also implies that certain experiences, particularly involving objectification of the body, become more likely (Bordo, 1993). Women have been shown to be significantly less satisfied with their bodies, due to a gender role which states that they must be beautiful and slender in order to attract a man, which should be of paramount importance in their lives. Even women of low body weight commonly diet, believing themselves fat. This becomes a problem when it is shown that these feelings of inadequacy about one's own body are linked to eating disorders, low self-esteem, depression, and lowered or insufficient use of contraceptives (Mintz and Betz, 1986). The role of sociocultural factors continues to be underemphasized in the theoretical and empirical literature and that the role of sociocultural influences needs to be closely examined.

Sex Roles and Gender Identity

Sex roles can be defined as a set of behaviors and characteristics that are standard for each gender in a society. Sex role stereotypes are widely-held beliefs about those behaviors and characteristics. Society forces people to adopt certain roles simply by expecting that those roles are proper and enforcing them.

Empirical findings support the view that sex roles are flexible and may be influenced by life situations and demands (Rewal and Kapur 1991). In general, the roles prevalent in modern Western society prescribe that men should be domineering, aggressive, and superior at mathematics and sciences, should become successful in their careers, and should control and suppress their feelings. Women, on the other hand, should be submissive, nurturing, gentle, better at languages and the humanities, emotional, and desirous of nothing more than a happy family and a husband to provide for her, while she remains at home and tends the house. These sex-typed roles are perpetuated and reinforced by the mass media and society in general in many ways, some obvious and others more subtle. Research conducted in the 1970s demonstrated that male and female psychologists listed the same ideal characteristics for a healthy "person" and a healthy "male", whereas their conception of a mature female was antithetical to their description of a healthy "person" (Broverman *et al*, 1972).

As described above, sex or gender roles are characteristics, behaviors and interests defined by a society or culture as appropriate for members of each sex. Many objective studies have found evidence linking gender traits to both problem eating and body dissatisfaction. Researchers have studied women with eating disorders, community and students samples consisting of young adult women and men, and adolescent girls and boys

(Murnen and Smolak, 1997). However, other kinds of relationships have also been found. Some empirical data suggest a relationship between low masculinity scores, problem eating, and body dissatisfaction (Holleran *et al*, 1988; Johnson *et al* 1996; Klingenspor, 1994). Some evidence supports that higher masculinity is associated with higher levels of problem eating (Cantrell and Ellis 1991; Silverstein *et al*, 1990). One study found that an undifferentiated gender personality, low feminine and low masculinity, was associated with problem eating in a clinical sample (Lewis and Johnson, 1985). Finally, another finding pointed out that lower femininity was associated with body dissatisfaction among a premenstrual group of adolescent girls whereas higher masculinity was associated with body dissatisfaction for menstrual girls (Usmiani and Daniluk, 1997).

Eating Disorders and Gender

Gender Differences and Disordered Eating

Women are remarkably more likely to develop eating disorders and their associated symptoms than men are (American Psychiatric Association, 2000). A variety of strong empirical evidence conducted since 1970 confirms that women perceive slenderness to be the most important aspect of physical attractiveness (Garner *et al*, 1985). The fact that young girls, but not young boys, have such precocious concerns about attractiveness is compelling evidence for the power of sex-role socialization and the potency of the diet message (Brumberg, 1988).

The onset of adolescence — the period of transition between childhood and adulthood — is usually accompanied by dramatic and often difficult changes in the life of a young person. Biological, cognitive, social, and environmental factors all contribute to influence an adolescent's personal development and self-esteem. Studies have shown that adolescent girls tend to have lower self-esteem and more negative assessments of their physical characteristics and intellectual abilities than boys have. These findings may explain why the incidence of suicide attempts, depression, and eating disorders is substantially higher in girls. Future research on methods for promoting self-esteem may help reduce the negative feelings of adolescent girls, as well as the problems that stem from them (Kearney-Cooke A, 1999).

In a large number of male and female college students, for males, the current ideal and attractive figures were near identical, and each was significantly more rounded than the average male figure preferred by women. That is, in general men misperceive the shape that appeals to women in a manner that reconciles it with their perception of their current shape and their ideal shape for themselves. It is very plausible that this "distortion" serves to maintain self-esteem (Lewinsohn *et al*, 1980). What a college woman thinks is attractive to men, however, is actually significantly thinner than the shape preferred by those men. Most important is the sad fact that the woman's ideal shape is even thinner than her misperception of the shape ideally attractive to men — in other words — it is the thinnest of all the ratings. Women's magazines may be particularly influential in the glorification of thinness, certainly contributing to the objectification of women, and to the reigning misbelief that to be fit is to be thin and *vice versa* (Garner *et al*, 1985).

The cultural deification of thinness has placed pressure on women to diet in order to conform to an unrealistic standard for feminine beauty. In puberty and adolescence a major portion of a young woman's weight gain derives from fat rather than muscle. While boys are developing muscles as a consequence of biological development, girls experience an increase in adiposity, particularly in their breasts and hips. In our fat phobic society, where female self-worth is so intimately tied to a slim figure, these biological differences have critical and distinctive emotional consequences. For adolescent boys, growing larger is frequently a source of pleasure and power; for girls, an increase in size is often confusing, awkward, and stressful. This distaste is expressed by many young girls through the wish to be thin; they no longer want to eat, they constantly watch their weight. In this sense, normal maturation in our society sets up young women for anorexia nervosa and/or bulimia nervosa.

Males and females are dissatisfied with different parts of their bodies. Most females are distressed about the areas below their waists, whereas males are more likely to be displeased with their upper bodies. More males that females would accept a normal body weight for age and height if they could choose a stereotypical male body image. Females, on the other hand, are more often motivated to attain a low body weight independent of shape. For most women raised in Western, industrialized nations, dieting is initiated as a result of a cultural endorsement of thinness (Vandereycken, 1992). In contrast, males who develop eating disorders begin dieting, in the majority of cases, (1) to avoid childhood teasing for being overweight; (2) to improve athletic performance; (3) to avoid developing medical illnesses associated with weight problems; and (4) to improve a homosexual relationship (Andersen and Holman, 1997). Unlike males, young women diet because of a common belief that weighing less is inherently good. In addition, males may also suffer from a relatively unknown form of eating disorder, "reverse anorexia", characterized by a fear of being thin and a drive for bulking up (Pope, 1993).

Moreover, Drewnowski and Yee (1987), Andersen and Holman (1997) have documented substantial gender differences with regard to perception of actual body weight as a percentage of a reference norm for age and height. According to these studies, adult women consider themselves thin at less than 87% of a healthy weight. Men however consider themselves thin up to 105% of a reference weight norm. The perception of being overweight is, therefore, highly dependent on gender. Furthermore, girls and young women appear to be more dedicated to the ideal of slimness than any religious, moral, or other social norm, whereas most males do not demonstrate a comparable preoccupation with body image.

It appears that gender differences emerge by middle school and possibly in elementary school (Smolak and Levine, 1994). Such gender differences have led theorists to attempt to tie gender role adoption to eating disorders. Hilde Bruch (1978) for example, suggested that anorexics might be trying to avoid female adulthood, particularly the reproductive and sexual aspects. Similarly, others have argued that bulimics are trying to reject the feminine, maternal roles ambivalently embraced by their stay-at-home-mothers (Silverstein and Perdue 1988).

On the other hand, Boskind-Lodahl (1976) proposed that women suffering from eating disorders were high in passivity, dependence, and need for approval from others (Morawsky, 1992). Steiner-Adair argued that the discrepancy between ideal and self-perceived masculine characteristics forms a basis for eating problems. More specifically, young women perceive that society values masculine characteristics, and so wish to possess them but fear they do not. They develop eating problems as a way of meeting the social demands for thinness, controlling their own bodies, and coping with the stress of their self-doubts. Thus, theoretical approaches vary dramatically in postulating relationships between traditionally defined gender roles (i.e., gender roles as measured by the Bem Sex Role Inventory (BSRI), Bem (1974) or the Personal Attributes Questionnaire (PAQ), (Spence and Helmreich, 1978) and eating disorders, especially anorexia nervosa and bulimia nervosa.

Sexual Orientation

Whereas male homosexuality is a risk factor for developing an eating disorder, lesbian orientation may be a protective factor, although this remains controversial (Siever, 1994). Approximately 20% of males suffering from eating disorders are homosexuals (Herzog *et al*, 1990). Gay men, who represent 3% to 5% of the total male population, exhibit a prevalence of eating disorders that is roughly four times greater than the total frequency of eating disorders. Male homosexuality is a risk factor for developing an eating disorder because of the increased value placed on thinness in the gay community compared with heterosexual environments (Siever, 1994).

One hundred university students (40 homosexual; 60 heterosexual) completed the Bem Sex Role Inventory and the Eating Attitudes Test. For the group as a whole, there were links between femininity and high levels of eating psychopathology, whereas masculinity was associated with relatively healthy eating-related attitudes and behaviours. When considering the role of sexual orientation, these links were specific to homosexual men and women. In relation to homosexual men and women, the results support a model where femininity might be seen as a specific risk factor for eating disorders, whereas masculinity is likely to be a protective factor (Meyer *et al*, 2001).

Siever (1994) confirmed the hypothesis that gay men and heterosexual women are dissatisfied with their bodies and vulnerable to eating disorders because of a shared emphasis on physical attractiveness and thinness, that is sustained on a desire to attract and please men. Although men place priority on physical attractiveness in evaluating potential partners, women place greater emphasis on other factors, such as personality, status, power, and income. Hence, lesbians and heterosexual men are less concerned with their own physical attractiveness and, consequently, less dissatisfied with their bodies and less vulnerable to eating disorders (Siever, 1994).

Femininity and Eating Disorders

In a meta-analytical review the relationship between femininity and eating disorders was based in 22 studies. Although the effect size was small it was significant, and showed that eating disordered women reported higher levels of femininity than non eating disordered women did (Murnen and Smolak, 1997). The largest effect size was found in the group of women diagnosed with anorexia nervosa. Eating disordered people had lower masculinity scores than did controls.

Females suffering from eating disorders are more likely to refuse traditional concepts of the female gender role, especially a traditional concept of motherhood (Henning K and Strauss B, 2003). When Steiner-Adair (1986), described "superwoman", a woman who achieves in both masculine (e.g., career, assertiveness) and feminine (e.g., family, nurturance) realms, and who is attractive while doing all of this, high schools girls who endorsed this image demonstrated greater eating pathology (Steiner Adair, 1986, 1989). Thorton and Leo (1991) reported similar findings for college women. Thus, "superwoman" may be a form of feminine gender role adoption which constitutes a risk factor for eating problems.

Silverstein and Perlick (1995) have suggested that it is the mismatch between an adolescent's modern gender role and her parents' traditional gender expectations that sets the stage for eating disorders. Thus far, the focus of gender eating disorders research has been on gender role adoption. However, being female means more than adopting a particular gender role. It also means that certain experiences, particularly involving objectification of the body, become more likely (Bordo, 1993). These experiences, including sexual harassment and sexual abuse, may be direct contributors to eating disorder (Wooley, 1994). Such experiences, especially when combined with society's sexual double standard, may leave young women confused about their sexual identity. Such confusion over society's messages and one's ability to control a sexual situation may lead to a sense of vulnerability, which may play out as an eating problem. The common finding that women suffering from bulimia nervosa are often promiscuous while those suffering from anorexia nervosa may appear to fear or be repulsed by sex suggests that sexual and eating issues are both body concerns for many women (Murnen and Smolak, 1997). Some developmentalists have suggested that early adolescence is a time of gender role shifts and gender intensification (e.g., Brown and Gilligan 1992). This is precisely the time that it appears to begin an intensification of eating problems in white American girls (Murnen and Smolak, 1997).

Relationship Between Eating Disorders and Gender Identity

The relationship between gender role and eating dysfunction is complex and requires multidimensional conceptualizations (Cantrell and Ellis, 1991).

Sociocultural pressures are divided into 3 categories; the thin ideal body for women, the centrality of appearance in the female gender role, and the importance of appearance for societal success. This model delineates probable carriers of cultural messages (peer, family, and media influences), examines relations between societal pressures and eating pathology, and considers the moderating role of internalizing societal pressures and of body dissatisfaction, restrained eating, negative affect, self-esteem and identity confusion, weight, social learning, coping skills, and impulsivity (Stice, 1994).

Internalization of sociocultural pressures mediate the adverse effects of the thin ideal. Stice *et al* (1994), found that our culture places a higher value on physical beauty in the evaluation of females than males. Garner *et al* (1980), have found that the average size of idealized woman (as portrayed by models), has become progressively thinner and has stabilized at 13% to19% below physically expected weight. Rodin *et al* (1984), suggest that this thin ideal is unachievable for most women and is likely to lead to feelings of self-devaluation, feelings of dysphoria (depression), and helplessness.

Feminine Gender Identity

Researchers and clinicians assert that there is an association between femininity and eating disorders, particularly anorexia nervosa and bulimia nervosa (Lancelot *et al*, 1994).

At present the relationship between eating disorders and feminine biology or sex role identity remains unclear; anorexia nervosa and bulimia have been variously associated with a rejection of femininity (Crisp, 1980), a confused acceptance of femininity (Boskind-White and White, 1983), and a rebellious redefinition of femininity (Orbach, 1985). These discrepancies in theory should not, however, obscure the obvious: the extreme sex difference in the prevalence of eating disorders means that the nature of femininity in our culture is a significant risk factor in the development of anorexia nervosa and bulimia.

Streigel-Moore *et al* (1986) discuss the relationship between eating disorders and many issues in the psychology of femininity, for example, the connections among physical attractiveness, pleasing and serving others, and self-esteem.

College women with bulimic behaviors tend to be more traditionally feminine in their sex-role identity and ideology than their nonbulimic peers (Brown *et al*, 1990). In a research, Szymanski and Chrisler (1990-91), observed that subjects that qualified in the feminine category on the Bem Sexual Role Inventory, ranged significantly higher on the Eating Disorders Inventory (EDI) (Garner *et al*, 1983) Bulimia subscale. Brown *et al* (1990), administering the Attitudes Scale and Personal Attributes Questionnaire, determined that a group of students with bulimic behaviors tended to be more traditionally feminine regarding her identity and ideology linked to sexual role than their non bulimic peers.

One of the explanations proposed for the "femininity hypothesis" is that the identification with characteristics typically labeled as "feminine", reflects a need of approval from others and lower self-esteem (Boskind-Lodahl, 1976; Paxton and Sculpthorpe, 1991). Data from sufferers of anorexia nervosa and bulimia nervosa are consistent with the presence of submissive behaviours and perceived low social rank (e.g. low self-esteem, helplessness, and feelings of shame). In a study, patients with eating disorders reported significantly higher levels of submissive behaviour and a more unfavourable social comparison than did student controls. Furthermore, levels of submissive behaviour and unfavourable social comparison were significantly related to severity of eating disorder symptoms, even after taking into account of depressive symptoms and other psychopathology (Troop *et al*, 2003).

Consequently, individuals who demonstrate higher levels of femininity are viewed as being more susceptible to the development of problem eating. Another possibility is that the relationship between femininity and problem eating for girls becomes more pronounced after adolescence and the onset of puberty. With the onset of puberty, girls experience a normative increase in body fat, which inevitably moves them further away from societal's ideal body shape for a woman. Therefore it is not surprising that several studies have found puberal development to be associated with higher levels of body dissatisfaction and disordered eating for girls (Attie and Brooks-Gunn, 1989; Swarr and Richards, 1996). In addition, during puberty adolescents receive greater pressures to conform to adult and gender roles (Alfieri *et al*, 1996; Basow 1992; Usmiani and Daniluk, 1997). Stereotypic behaviors and attitudes as reflected by gender traits are likely to play a more important role in determining psychological adjustment and problem eating. Further research is needed to examine how the development of puberty may moderate the relationship between femininity and disordered eating among adolescent girls. (Thomas and Ricciardelli, 2000)

Overall, the array of findings suggests that there may be more than one dimension underlying the relationship between gender traits, problem eating, and body dissatisfaction (Davis *et al*, 1996). Therefore, further research is needed to help us clarify the nature and the development of the relationship.

PSYCHOSOCIAL PROFILE OF EATING DISORDERED WOMEN

Current theorists have also suggested that gender role orientation, self-esteem, and dependence on others' approval are associated with disordered eating. Those who have addressed gender role orientation have claimed that either extreme femininity (Boskind-Lodahl 1976; Boskind-White and White, 1983; Bruch, 1978) or rejection of femininity (Chernin 1985; Orbach 1978; Thomä, 1967) is found in disordered eating. Related to the need for approval is the suggestion that both anorexics (Crisp, 1980) and bulimics (Boskind-Lodahl, *et al*, 1978; Hawkins and Clement, 1984) exhibit low self-confidence and self-esteem. A uniform picture has emerged of the eating disordered woman as a dependent, immature, "good girl" with an "abnormal" gender role identity (Beren and Chrisler, 1990).

Wilson, White (1946) and Crisp (1967, 1977) concluded that immaturity is integrally related to the eating disorder. Some researchers suggest that bulimics are "hyperfeminine" (Boskind-Lodhal 1976; Boskind-Lodhal *et al*, 1978) or they are more likely than non disordered eaters to endorse the traditional feminine role (Rost *et al*, 1982). Lewis and Johnson (1985) compared scores on the Bem Sex Roles Inventory for a group of bulimic women and a non-disordered control group and found that a significant number of bulimics were classified as undifferentiated. The authors conclude that bulimics may not have a clearly defined sense of self and suggest that this undifferentiated orientation may reflect a different type of feminine identification, as women have traditionally been socialized away from self-identification through others. These results support Chernin's (1985) theory that eating disordered women lack a sense of identity. A significant number of eating disordered women did describe themselves as childlike on the Bem Sex Role Inventory; a finding that may actually relate to the eating disordered women's lack of self-esteem, in that they do not perceive themselves as capable and adult-like because they are not confident in their abilities. In our society men are judged by the qualities of their minds, women are judged by the qualities of their bodies (Freedman 1986; Greenspan 1983). Women think that they must be attractive, and, today that means being thin. Eating disordered women, with their low self-confidence and self-esteem, would be especially susceptible to these sociocultural pressures. Because of this lack of self-esteem, thinness may assume a key importance as they overemphasize its necessity and believe that once they become thin (and hence attractive) that they will also be happy, successful, and confident (Boskind-White and White, 1983).

Boskind-White and White (1983), point out that these young women are generally bright, energetic, talented, interesting, and privileged. But this potential only seems to contribute to a strong feeling of being trapped between a dedication to traditional feminine values and an overpowering sense that they must compete with men and women in developing a successful career. To maintain the balance of power in favor of men or some vague conception of the *status quo*, this resistant majority has perverted the feminist demands for equality of opportunity into an unrealistic insistence that women reconcile the traditional and contradictory masculine and feminine roles into a "super" identity (Boskind-White, 1983). This identity retains many features of the established feminine role, for example, an obsession with the body, sensitivity to others, and dependence on male approval, but redefines the substance and style of femininity to emphasize thinness, youth, ambition, self-control, and self-sufficiency (Boskind-White, 1985).

Moreover, it is likely that rejection of the stereotypical feminine role with its images of a soft, rounded, and self-effacing mother contributes in some way to our cultural obsession with thinness (Garner *et al*, 1983). The other side of the new coin may be the need to look younger and more masculine, that is, thinner, in order to compete and gain respect in the essentially masculine world of business. Or both motives can be condensed into a single need, to compete with other women over who is the thinnest and most virtuous at the dinner table. The new, slender style is not a true symbol of liberation, but simply a newer badge of subjugation, this time to a god of thinness that is much more dangerous than whalebone corsets or stiletto heels (Boskind-White, 1985).

Steiner-Adair found that of all the girls attending a private high school, a group at risk for eating disorders, was quite aware of the "superwoman" ideal. These girls were able to describe themselves as thin, attractive, smart, active, independent, autonomous, and dominant within relationships, and somehow perfectly successful in establishing a career, being an exciting wife, and raising a family. Sixty percent of the girls seemed to understand that pursuing this myth would jeopardize the sense of interpersonal connectedness around which girls, as opposed to boys, tend to build their identities (Gilligan C, 1982). Forty percent wholeheartedly embraced this contradictory vision of interdependent autonomy, seeing no internal inconsistencies and no dissonance between the intense pressure to be separate *versus* their socialization to value relationship above complete individuation. Of the girls who saw through the superwoman myth and rejected it, not one had an Eating Attitudes Test (EAT) (Garner *et al*, 1982) score in the eating disorder range. Of the girls who identified themselves with the superwoman, 85% had scores in the eating disorder range and another one was borderline. Levine (1987) assumes that the work of Boskind-White and Steiner-Adair provides strong support for the belief that complex transformations in the feminine role constitute a sociocultural factor in the proliferation of eating disorders.

Maternal Identification

Very few of today's women feel that their mothers like their own bodies. Additionally, a woman's negative attitude toward her own body is highly correlated with the perception that both the mother and the father are or were critical of her body shape. Levine (1987) and Wooley and Wooley (1985) point out that the mothers of today's teenage girls are the first cohort of women to experience generalized dissatisfaction with their weight and themselves as a result of fashion propaganda, the changing roles of women, and our culture's increasing emphasis on youth. When these girls reach puberty, or even before, their body shape may become a projective surface for their mother's unfulfilled wishes and uncertainties and for the daughter's needs to act like a woman (mother) while becoming her own, "better" woman (not mother). In this emotionally charged interaction, dieting may serve simultaneously as identification, differentiation, revenge, and penance. Perhaps the hostile purification of the anorexic and the uncontrollable gorging and purging of the bulimic represent a culturally supported lack of respect for the normal female body and a need to escape the choices posed by the dilemma of maternal *versus* paternal identification.

The Role of the Feminist Movement

The proliferation of eating disorders has coincided, not only with feminism and increasing pressures for thinness, but also with an explosion of violence against women in the streets, at home, on films, and in literature. Surely such denigration does nothing to help girls and women learn how to respect their bodies and themselves. Furthermore, women are socialized to deny anger or keep it to themselves. Both these factors increase the likelihood that eating disorders are in part self-directed expressions of rage that also serve to mock the very same dependency, objectification, and idealization of thinness that many anorexics and bulimics cannot refrain from embodying. Now many vulnerable people, young women, convert powerful new conflicts between internal needs (to "be in control" and to "be someone") and external properties ("being thin" and "feminine") into eating disorders.

Wooley and Wooley (1985) propose three facts that clearly connect eating disorders with changes in the feminine sex role. First, the upsurge of eating disorders coincides with the increased impact of the feminist movement and the resultant expansion of the feminine sex role to include contradictory demands for autonomous and interdependent behaviors. Second, most anorexics and bulimics are female who develop their eating disorders during adolescence, a time of life in which issues of identity and intimacy are paramount in personal development. Third, the research by Steiner-Adair demonstrates a correlation between identification with the "super-thin superwoman" ideal and anorexic-like attitudes and behaviors. At present we do not know precisely how these confusing and oppressive changes in the feminine sex role combine with the traditional feminine investment in personal appearance to set the stage for eating disorders. It is very likely, however that the relentless pursuit of thinness reflects numerous themes, including identification with current ideals of youthful beauty, rejection of traditional feminine shapes and limitations, and the struggle for control of something concrete – weight and shape – in a world of abstract ambiguities. (Wooley and Wooley, 1985; Orbach, 1985; Boskind-White, 1985).

Schwartz *et al* (1982) believe that rather the association between the feminist movement and eating disorders, this fact may indicate "if one lives in a culture where the roles of women are complex, conflicting, and in change, and these pressures exist in a milieu which emphasizes a high positive value on slimness and negative value on obesity, one is at greater risk for anorexia (and bulimia).

A Feminist View

The emphasis on feminine attractiveness has continued despite the changing social roles, expectations, and opportunities for women that have occurred in the past 30 years or so. Moreover, these social changes have contributed to increase stress for women resulting from conflict between many of the competing role demands, facing them in both personal and professional aspects of their lives (Emmett 1985; Orbach 1978, 1986; Palazzoli, 1978).

Feminists see the expectation that a woman be physically attractive and capable of being an effective wife, mother, and working woman as an ideal that many women attempt to achieve, yet frequently find to be unrealistic, unattainable, undesirable, and oppressive (Orbach, 1978).

According to Orbach (1978), being fat or eating compulsively is a directed conscious or unconscious challenge to sex-role stereotyping and the culturally defined experience of womanhood. In other words, a woman is expected by society to market herself as being available to men, marriage and motherhood. In the face of this pressure, exploited by advertising and the media, her desire to realize her potential as a person becomes of secondary importance in relation to her public image as an attractive female package. For some women compulsive eating develops as a way to avoid being "marketed" in this way, a way to avoid competition with other women, and possibly the only way for a woman to defend herself against the powerlessness of her position in society *vis-à-vis* men (Gilbert S, 1986).

It is suggested that disordered eating reflects women's response to the stress of these multiple pressures and conflicting demands (Orbach, 1978; Palazzoli, 1978). Thus, in a culture in which women's roles are complex and frequently conflicting, and the emphasis placed on appearance and thinness results in unrealistic body image and body dissatisfaction, conditions exist for heightened chronic stress and reduced self-esteem that may contribute to increased risk among women of developing an eating disorder (Schwartz *et al*, 1985).

There is the argument, on the one hand, that the female role makes women vulnerable to coercion, whereas on the other, it is seen as the source of women's personal conflict. A feminist perspective tends to emphasize the coercive elements in the female role. Women, it is argued, generally have much less control over their lives than men, and they are also subject to the quite explicit expectation that they should conform to a stereotypical body shape. The requirement is that they should be thin. This expectation is coercive, for the cost of failing to conform to conventional standards of slimness is to be made to feel unacceptable. There are many who are likely to be particularly vulnerable to such pressures during adolescence. There is the rather more subtle idea that emaciation and obesity are alternative strategies which enable women to escape from the demands of their role. By being either too fat or too thin a woman avoids being an object of sexual attraction. Being "outside the status of sex object" the anorexic is thus refusing to fit in with the expectation that she should be passive, decorative and dependent, and in so doing she is daring to define herself. The anorexic's modification of her body shape, like that of the obese woman, is an attempt to establish her existence as an individual independent of her female role, in so far as the emaciation in the anorexic will eventually produce physical weakness and with this a state of greater ineffectiveness and so dependence (Orbach S, 1978).

Feminists, often therapists, avoid casting the eating disordered behaviour as pathological. Instead, they seek to demonstrate that these disorders are an inevitable consequence of a misogynistic society that demeans women by devaluing female experience and women's values, by objectifying their bodies, and by discrediting vast areas of women's past and present achievements. Both overeating and noneating are a "protest against the way in which women are regarded in our society as objects of adornment and pleasure" (Orbach, 1986).

Boskind-White and White (1983) and Boskind-Lodahl (1976) suggest that the most appropriate treatment for anorexia nervosa and bulimia should include feminist therapy, which emphasizes the sociocultural influences which shape eating disorders and which recognizes the importance of increasing the disordered eaters' self-esteem, self-control, and feelings of empowerment.

The Influence of Gender Role in the Development

Some degree of conflict is inherent in the female roles. All the child needs to develop an adequate role concept that comes from experience of the wider culture. At a wider social and cultural level the girl is confronted with a scale that stresses the worth and importance of assertiveness, independence, intellectual prowess, the ability to be productive, and other attributes of this kind which are aligned far more with the role requirements for boys than with those for her own sex. They are attributes that have a positive value in general social terms, but a negative value for the girl in terms of her female role. This requires that she should be passive, yielding and dependent, decorative rather than productive, and helpless rather than competent. Such attributes as these conflicts rather than coincide with wider social values. Then, it is not surprising, that even at quite an early age there is evidence that the self esteem of boys is markedly higher than the self-esteem of girls (Kohlberg, 1966).

Although the educational system ostensibly prepares and encourages men and women equally for higher education and careers, these are really limited by both social and psychological pressures to men. While decrying the loss of female potential in both economic and personal terms, society provides little, if any, positive encouragement for women to be interested in pursuing a career. The culturally prevalent view is that femininity and individual achievement are mutually exclusive ends. Female students clearly associate unusual academic excellence in women with loss of femininity, social rejection and "personal and societal destruction". Some have stressed that it means that a woman could be unhappy, aggressive, and unmarried. It is at puberty that the "motive to avoid success" emerges, when there is an increased awareness of gender roles and the tendency to be particularly vulnerable to social ostracism. From this time onwards a girl is likely to experience anxiety in relation to her role. Anxiety is also experienced most frequently when women compete with men in traditionally male-dominated areas. It is believed that fear of success is largely responsible for the substantial under representation of women in higher education. Certainly some women do overcome many of the pressures and pursue a career, but few manage this without feeling guilty, anxious, unfeminine, and selfish (Slade, 1984).

From earliest childhood men learn that their role is to be active, intelligent, dominant, rational, and assertive. Women learn at a similarly early age that assertiveness on their part is inappropriate; taking initiative is not their task. Their concern is with caring and nurturing, with being receptive to the feelings of those around them, with being sensitive and supportive in their response to human needs. Not only does this strength and competence often go unrecognized and unacknowledged but, it is all too likely to be systematically devalued. And at best it is represented as feminine weakness, and at worst as female pathology. Women all too often fulfill the demands of their female role to the best of their ability, deriving meanwhile precious little self-esteem from their endeavours. Furthermore, the particular concerns that their role assigns to them gives them greater experience generally in human development and personal relationships. Women, learn to judge themselves in the same way as they are judged by the dominant culture. This contributes to her sense of unworthiness and to her feeling that she is being given help and resources that she does not deserve, and often which the family cannot easily afford (Slade, 1984).

The Influence of the Family as Predisposing Factor

The eating disordered patients, particularly the anorexic feels she is under strong pressure to succeed educationally, and to pursue a career. Her family is all the more pleased when her career is one that carries high status, which often means that she is competing, or preparing to compete, in male-dominated professions.

The anorexic shares with her family a powerful ethic of individual effort and self-improvement. Anorexic's families are generally concerned with social position, respectability, and financial security. Success is important to them. In this context being emotional and expressing feelings is far from a priority. There is less demand upon women to control or repress their feelings. As a consequence they, far more than men, become familiar with their feelings and obtain openness in dealing with them. The fact which is generally overlooked in psychological accounts of anorexia nervosa is that this kind of emotionally supportive response is entirely compatible with the requirements of the female role. The anorexic's response to her parents' needs may indicate her "abnormal considerateness", even her "over submissiveness". It is this receptivity to human needs as a characteristic of the female role that provides the link between the anorexic and the values and experiences of her family. As a result of her upbringing – in the widest possible sense – the anorexic becomes attuned to responding to the needs of those around her: to being sensitive, compliant, supportive, and making others feel at ease; she is so attuned because she is female. Moreover, receptivity is a personal attribute which she herself values (Slade, 1984).

Gender roles indicate to the individual a way of ordering priorities. The anorexic is quite unable to decide, however, whether being sensitive to others should take precedence over the performance of the task, or *vice versa*. The anorexic cannot easily order her priorities because she feels obliged to respond both in a way that is generally considered socially desirable for males, and in a way that is considered socially desirable for females. It is, paradoxically, because of her female receptivity that she feels obliged take on the male tasks of being a good performer and achiever of success. Her family's values create the obligation for its members to respond in ways that are valued for males, but this is only possible, and can only be maintained, through their being aware and receptive in a way that is valued for females.

What is in fact taking place between the anorexic and her family is a skewed transaction. Her parents see her as developing intellectual potential and as being given every encouragement to make something of herself, and, having her best interests at heart, they provide her with opportunities that they probably had to strive for, and which her grandparents may never have had. The anorexic, meanwhile, being sensitive to her parents' values and attitudes, knows that achievement will please them and sees it as her task to be successful, even though she feels unequal to this. Through her success and her loyalty in this respect, she helps to underpin her family's sense of establishment and well-being. However, she places no particular value for herself on what is involved in doing good. Her family praises her for her success, but they fail to acknowledge this contribution to their feeling of well-being for the service that it is. The praises the girl receives she feels are empty, for being told how good she is for doing something she does not value does nothing to increase her own sense of worth. As in all such skewed transactions the anorexic is left with the overall feeling that she is "bad" (Slade, 1984).

SANDRA BEM AND SEX ROLES CATEGORIES

The Concept of Androgyny

As previously mentioned, there is a consensus on the stereotyped roles for the average man or woman. The traits in these stereotypes fall into two separate groups. The first expresses competence and independence, while the second focuses on warmth and expressiveness. Men are seen as having the competence, while women are seen as more expressive. Some of these traits are: feminine (tactful, quiet, aware of feelings of others, need for security, easily express tender feeling), masculine (aggressive, independent, dominant, competitive, active, ambitious, make decisions easily). Competence (masculine) traits are valued more in Western societies; in contrast expressive (feminine) traits are viewed negatively.

Sandra Lipsitz Bem, a Stanford University psychologist, introduced the concept of androgyny (1977) that seeks to indicate the degree to which a person is culturally influenced by gender roles. This word comes from the Greek: *andro* for male and *gyne* for female referring to a blending of what are usually agreed as positive characteristics of both sexes. The androgynous individual possesses flexibility. S/he can be assertive, independent, and self-reliant as well as relate to others, be sensitive to others' needs, and is able to depend on others for emotional support. Androgyny allows an individual to be independent and tender, assertive and yielding, masculine and feminine. Thus androgyny greatly expands the range of behavior open to everyone, permitting people to cope more effectively with diverse situations as well as assimilate the understanding necessary to develop mature, lasting relationships. The androgynous person is high in both masculine and feminine traits. Bem hypothesized that psychological androgyny with equally high levels of feminine and masculine traits constitute optimal mental health for both men and women. She also argued that masculinity and femininity were independent dimensions, with the possibility of both sets of characteristics co-existing in the one individual. Androgynous people can be aggressive or yielding, forceful or gentle, sensitive or assertive, as the particular situation requires. Likewise, feminine women have trouble being independent and assertive, even when independence and assertiveness are needed. In contrast, choosing from a wider range of behaviors, truly androgynous people are able to modify their responses, according to their needs and the needs of the situation. Bem believed that androgynous people are freer, more adaptable, and more emotionally healthy than those who restrict their behavior to traditional sex roles.

Bem Sex Role Inventory (Bem 1974) consists of 60 self-descriptive, personality-characteristic adjectives designed to measure psychological masculinity and femininity as two independent variables. All adjectives are designed to be positive toned, or socially desirable. This scale is measuring the cultural, not biological influences on gender roles. Twenty items assess masculinity, 20 assess femininity, the others are neutral. Each adjective is ranked on a Likert scale where 1= 'never or almost never true' and 7= 'always or almost always true'. Scores on each dimension can range from 20 to 140. Individuals are classified on the basis of median splits as 'masculine' (high masculinity, low femininity), 'feminine' (high femininity, low masculinity), 'androgynous' (high masculinity and femininity), or 'undifferentiated' (low masculinity and femininity) and contains a 10-item masculinity and a 10 item femininity scale. In determining a person's sex-role on this scale, the medians of masculinity and femininity scales are derived. Individuals who score above both medians are androgynous, while people scoring below both medians are considered undifferentiated. A man who scores above the median on the masculinity scale and below the median on the femininity scale is a traditional male, and a woman who scores below the masculinity but above the femininity median display a traditional feminine sex-role.

Gender Stereotyped Traits in Eating Disordered Patients

Gender traits, typically referred to as "masculinity and "femininity", provide one of the ways for studying the sociocultural context underlying many of our attitudes and behaviors. Specifically gender traits reflect stereotypes about the beliefs and behaviors typically attributed to men and women, which are acquired as they learn about the world and their roles in it (Basow, 1992; Deux and Major, 1987).

The presence of sex role stereotypes in the population as a whole has been demonstrated many times (Slade, 1984). The author describes one study in which a large sample of men and women was presented with a list of personal characteristics and asked how desirable they, as individuals, felt it was for men and for women in society to have these characteristics. Both men and women decided that certain characteristics — such as forceful, analytical, ambitious — were socially desirable for men, whereas other characteristics — such as affectionate, yielding, sensitive to the needs of others — were socially desirable for women. Other characteristics such as truthful and happy were judged to be equally desirable for men and women, and were therefore placed in a neutral category that make possible to identify individuals who accept that they have characteristics that are socially desirable for males and for females. Anorexics were generally more satisfied with themselves in relation to stereotypically female characteristics than stereotypically male characteristics; they were more satisfied particularly in relation to those female characteristics associated with sensitivity to other people. The socially desirable characteristics for females that they considered important to decision making were loyalty, sympathy, sensitivity to the needs of others, and understanding. They rejected all other feminine characteristics, and this included such attributes as warm, yielding, affectionate, and tender. Of those traits socially desirable for males, they accepted analytical, independent, self-reliant and, for obvious reasons, the ability to make decisions easily, as being important to this task. Among the other male-valued characteristics that they rejected were such attributes as aggressive, competitive, having a strong personality, and willingness to take a stand. Many neutral qualities were accepted as important to decision making as both male and female qualities together. In other words, faced with the problem of having to make up her mind what to do in any situation, the anorexic is the more likely to attempt to be adaptable, sincere, helpful, reliable, truthful, and conscientious; thus choosing to avoid, where possible, gender type characteristics. Likewise the anorexic values certain aspects of the female role whilst strenuously rejecting others. Sympathy, sensitivity, and understanding are most important to her, but the openness and spontaneity of feeling that are usually accepted as accompanying these qualities, and as essential to their normal expression, are given no part in her life. The emotionality that is implicit in such female characteristics as tender, warm, affectionate, love for children, she has learned to reject. Thus, within the female role too she is taking on the task of being sensitive and responding to the needs of those around her without assuming those aspects of the role that will enable her to perform those tasks more fully and with greater personal satisfaction. She is acutely sensitive to other people's feelings; she is also utterly convinced that she must keep her own feelings to herself. Her sense of failure and accumulating feelings of inadequacy are aspects of her life that she must not burden anyone with, least of all members of her family. Anorexic's families generally maintain the inherent contradiction of negating the value of feelings while demanding sensitivity to the need for loyalty and cohesion; the situation is further complicated by their ambivalence towards other kinds of behaviour which conventionally belong to the female role (Slade, 1984; Behar, 1992).

Behar *et al* (2001) compared female eating disordered patients *versus* female university students without eating problems and confirmed that the feminine condition emerges as the main category of gender identity in the formers, whilst healthy students were mainly identified with androgyny category. Eating disordered patients displayed the following profile on BSRI: childlike, moody, willing to take a stand, unpredictable, jealous, conventional, and inefficient. These traits are according with clinical characteristics widely seen among anorexics and bulimics. In contrast, female students without eating dysfunctions were more sympathetic, happy, self-reliant, independent, and assertive, made decisions easily, self-sufficient, helpful, conscientious, truthful, gentle, and tactful. These predominant neutral traits are protective, beneficial, adaptable, favorable, and determinant to obtain a desirable and ideal biopsychosocial welfare. Feminine characteristics such as loyalty, femininity, understanding, sensitivity to other's needs, were sociably desirable for eating disordered subjects; masculine traits such as defends own beliefs, willing to take a stand, analytical, and independent, were more valued by them, and among neutral features, they preferred to be reliable, sincere, friendly, and secretive. In this research, a 42.9% of the patients, in contrast with the 23.8% of the students were classified within the Feminine category. Contrary, a 31.7% and a 42.9% of the latter was qualified as Androgynous and Undifferentiated *versus* the 19% and 27% of the patients respectively. There were significant differences between patients and students in 22 items of the BSRI ($p < 0.01$). Both groups rejected and were identified with some feminine, masculine and neutral qualities (table 1).

In another analyses, Behar *et al* (2002) confronted female eating disordered patients *versus* non clinical populations of female and male subjects without eating problems corroborating their earlier results and demonstrating that female subjects without eating disorders showed more drive for thinness and displayed more body dissatisfaction than their male peers (tables 2 and 3).

Additionally, they found (2003) the highest percentage of feminine category on the BSRI among restricted anorexics, and simultaneously they ranked higher on the EDI Maturity fears subscale. Again, femininity emerged as the main trait of gender identity in patients suffering from an eating pathology, in contrast to androgyny showed by female subjects without eating disorders (figure 1). Restrictive anorectics displayed more femininity than the others eating disorders subtypes. Compulsive.purgative anorectics showed more level of severity within the eating disorder spectrum, and more drive for thinness, perfectionism and interpersonal distrust. Restrictive anorectics exhibited more maturity fears and purgative bulimics more bulimic behaviours, body dissatisfaction, ineffectiveness and interoceptive awareness (figures 2 and 3).

Table 1. Comparison of answers on the BRSI between groups TCA (N= 63) y C (N= 63)

Item	Category	ED Group		E Group		p Val
		X	DE	X	DE	
Cheerful (B5)	Feminine	5,0	(1,6)	5,9	(0,8)	<0,001*
Sympathetic (B23)	Feminine	5,0	(1,7)	6,2	(0,6)	<0,001*
Childlike (B50)	Feminine	4,3	(1,8)	3,0	(1,4)	<0,001*
Self-reliant	Masculine	4,4	(1,8)	6,0	(0,9)	<0,001* (B1)
Independent (B7)	Masculine	5,0	(1,7)	5,9	(1,0)	<0,001*
Assertive (B13)	Masculine	4,6	(1,7)	5,6	(0,9)	<0,001*
Analytical (B22)	Masculine	5,3	(1,8)	6,0	(1,0)	0,008*
Makes decisions easily (B31)	Masculine	3,8	(1,8)	5,1	(1,2)	<0,001*
Self-sufficient (B34)	Masculine	4,6	(1,9)	5,8	(1,0)	<0,001*
Willing to take a position (B43)	Masculine	5,6	(1,7)	4,0	(1,7)	<0,001*
Helpful (B3)	Neutral	4,8	(1,7)	6,0	(0,9)	<0,001*
Moody (B6)	Neutral	5,3	(1,8)	3,7	(1,9)	<0,001*
Conscientious (B9)	Neutral	5,4	(1,5)	6,3	(1,0)	<0,001*
Happy (B15)	Neutral	4,2	(1,7)	6,0	(0,9)	<0,001*
Unpredictable (B18)	Neutral	4,7	(1,8)	3,7	(1,6)	<0,001*
Jealous (B24)	Neutral	5,0	(1,8)	4,4	(1,8)	0,047*
Truthful (B27)	Neutral	5,4	(1,7)	6,2	(0,7)	<0,001*
Sincere (B33)	Neutral	6,1	(1,1)	6,4	(0,6)	0,021*
Likable (B39)	Neutral	5,4	(1,2)	5,9	(0,7)	0,003*
Solemn (B42)	Neutral	4,3	(1,7)	3,3	(1,4)	<0,001*
Inefficient (B48)	Neutral	2,9	(1,6)	1,9	(1,1)	<0,001*
Tactful (B57)	Neutral	5,1	(1,8)	5,7	(0,8)	0,017*

X = Mean   ED group = Eating disordered patients
DE = Standard deviation   E Group = Students without eating problems
* = Statistically significant difference

The distinction between anorexia nervosa and bulimia is often not well defined, they frequently co-occur, and both may be symptomatic of common antecedents (Hsu, 1990). Related to the need for approval is the suggestion that both anorexics (Crisp, 1980) and bulimics (Boskind-Lodahl, Sirlin and White, 1978; Hawkins and Clement, 1984) have low self-confidence and self- esteem. People classified as undifferentiated on the Bem Sex Role Inventory have also been found to report significantly lower self-esteem, as measured by the Texas Social Behavior Inventory, than androgynous, masculine, or feminine subjects (Bem, 1977; Lewis and Johnson, 1985, Spence, Helmreich and Stapp, 1975). Lewis and Johnson (1985) reported bulimics to be less feminine than control subjects; Katzman and Wolchik (1984), however, reported no differences in femininity or masculinity between bulimics and controls. Anorexics, on the other hand, reportedly do not differ from control subjects on femininity, but are less masculine than controls (Sitnick and Katz, 1984). Murnen and Smolak

(1996) in their meta-analysis, found the largest effect size in the group of women diagnosed with anorexia nervosa that were likely to score higher on the gender role assures compared to control groups. In nineteen of the studies, eating disordered people had lower masculinity scores than did controls (Murnen and Smolak, 1996).

Table 2. Comparison of variables between groups TCA (n= 119) y F (n= 63)

Variable	ED Group		F Group		p Value
	$\bar{X}$	DE	$\bar{X}$	DE	
Present weight	54,9	(10,7)	55,8	(5,8)	NS
Height	157,7	(21,4)	161,3	(5,3)	NS
Ideal weight	50,5	(5,7)	53,5	(4,7)	<0,001*
EAT-40	51,6	(21,4)	10,4	(6,4)	<0,001*
EDI	87,6	(31,6)	23,3	(18,2)	<0,001*
Drive for thinness	14,4	(6,3)	2,4	(3,9)	<0,001*
Interoceptive awareness	13,3	(6,9)	1,1	(2,6)	<0,001*
Bulimia	8,8	(5,8)	2,5	(1,9)	<0,001*
Body dissatisfaction	15,8	(8,1)	5,1	(6,6)	<0,001*
Ineffectiveness	9,0	(7,6)	0,9	(2,0)	<0,001*
Maturity fears	11,1	(6,1)	3,9	(4,2)	<0,001*
Perfectionism	9,2	(4,3)	6,2	(4,4)	<0,001*
Interpersonal distrust	6,0	(5,2)	1,3	(2,0)	<0,001*

X = Mean ED group = Eating disordered subjects
DE = Standard deviation F group = Female students without eating problems
* = Statistically significant difference
NS = No significant difference

Table 3. Comparison of variables between M (n= 89) and F (n= 63) groups

Variable	M Group		F Group		p Value
	$\bar{X}$	DE	$\bar{X}$	DE	
Present weight	73,7	(9,7)	55,8	(6,0)	<0,001*
Height	176,2	(7,1)	161,3	(5,3)	<0,001*
Ideal weight	72,6	(8,4)	53,5	(4,7)	<0,001*
EAT-40	10,7	(5,8)	10,4	(6,4)	NS
EDI	21,7	(11,6)	23,3	(18,3)	NS
Drive for thinness	0,9	(2,1)	2,4	(3,9)	0,003*
Interoceptive awareness	1,2	(1,8)	1,1	(2,6)	NS
Bulimia	2,4	(1,7)	2,5	(1,9)	NS
Body dissatisfaction	2,8	(3,9)	5,1	(6,6)	0,009*
Ineffectiveness	0,6	(1,4)	0,9	(2,0)	NS
Maturity fears	3,9	(3,9)	3,9	(4,2)	NS
Perfectionism	7,7	(3,5)	6,2	(4,4)	0,020*
Interpersonal distrust	2,3	(2,4)	1,3	(2,0)	0,008*

X = Mean ED group = Eating disordered subjects
DE = Standard deviation F group = Male students without eating problems
* = Statistically significant difference
NS = No significant difference

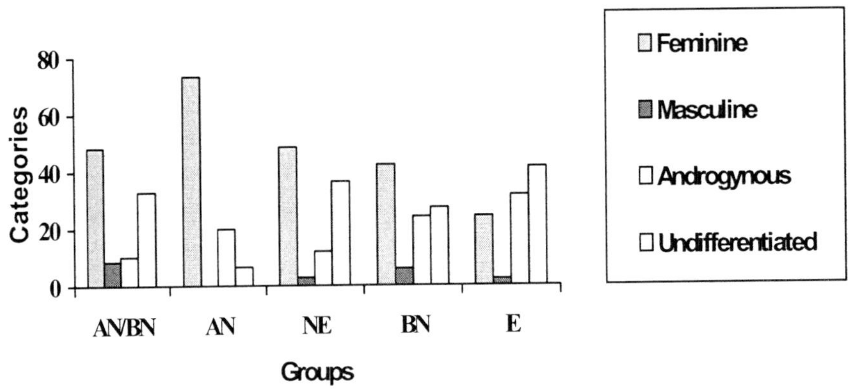

Figure 1. Gender identity categories on the BRSI and its difference among groups.

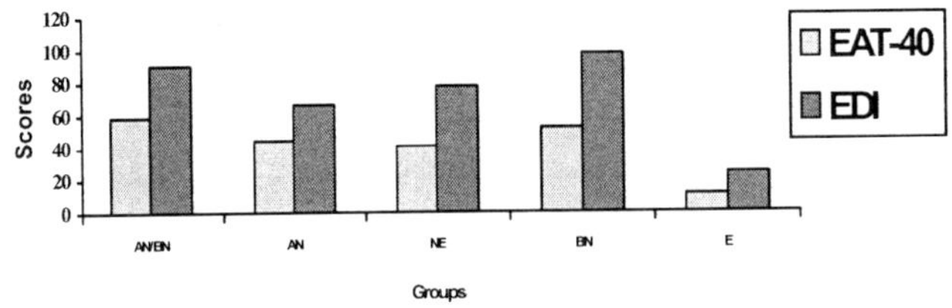

Figure 2. EAT-40 and EDI scores among groups.

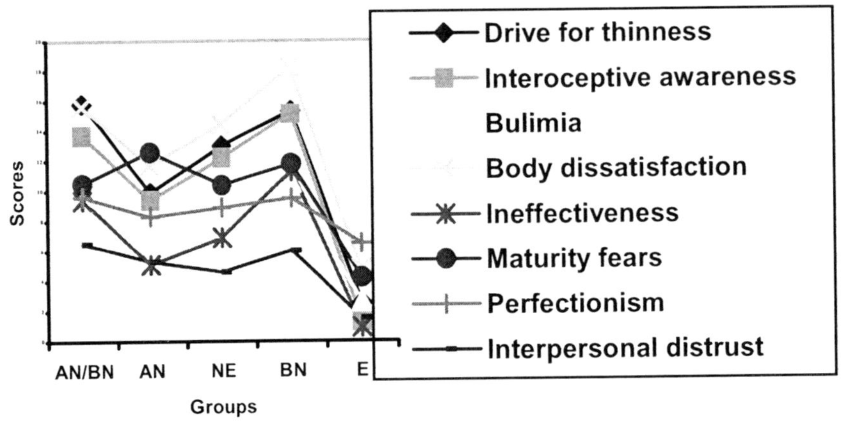

Figure 3. EDI scores and its items among groups.

Evidence About Androgyny

There is a growing evidence in the literature regarding androgynous traits.

Androgynous approaches promise increased independent thinking, action, and self-esteem, (Bradley, 1993; Shimonaka *et al*, 1994) and androgynous people prefer other androgynous people (Orlofsky, 1982; Pursell, *et al*, 1981).

Throughout life span of both sexes, it has been found that there is a relationship between androgyny and successful adaptation. Self-esteem and subjective health seems to be the most effective predictors of adaptation. (Shimonaka *et al*, 1997) In fact, scores on a measure of androgyny are predictive of those on an index of empathy in medical students and residents (Yarnold *et al*, 1993).

On the other hand, Napholz (1994) observed that subjects who were undifferentiated in sex role orientation had significantly higher depression scores, lower self-esteem scores, and lower life satisfaction scores than the androgynous and cross-typed groups. Androgyny is an instance of a more general situational flexibility (Vonk and Ashmore, 1993), and is associated with more liberal attitudes toward sexual expression (Johnson, 1989). In a study, participants high on androgyny reported less same sex and opposite sex touch avoidance than did subjects low on androgyny (Crawford, 1994); is predictive of greater life satisfaction than an undifferentiated orientation (Dean and Gilroy, 1993), is related to characteristics that enhance the development and maintenance of close friendships, such as a communal orientation and positive conceptions of friends (Jones *et al*, 1990). On the other hand, androgynous profiles are rated as more desirable across occupations (Arkkelin and O'Connor, 1992). Androgynous nurses reported lower depression and vocational stress than their undifferentiated counterparts (Steenbarger and Greenberg, 1990).

Androgynous and undifferentiated women may possess specific characteristics that enable them to cope effectively with the different and conflicting demands of masculine and feminine roles. In addition (Root, 1990) notes certain other "protective factors" with regard to disordered eating (high self-esteem, emotional stability, low self-consciousness, and an emphasis on healthy body rather than appearance) that may be more characteristic of androgynous women; for instance, androgynous individuals have the highest levels of self-esteem among the four gender categories and undifferentiated individuals typically have the lowest self-esteem (Bem 1977; Spence and Helmreich, 1978) as well as generally lower achievement motivation (Spence, Helmreich, 1978).

Hypothesis concerning the relationship of sex role flexibility (androgyny) to mental health have been supported for females in both college and psychiatric populations (Burchardt and Serbin, 1982). Highly feminine women are more likely to have weak body boundaries than more androgynous women (Ricards and McAlister, 1994). In light of a society not yet gender schematic, psychological androgyny is invoked as the development ideal (Mead and Ignico, 1992).

Finally, Skoe (1995) described that high levels of care-based moral reasoning, i.e., a balanced concern for the welfare of self and others, was related to androgyny for women. According to this author, women in particular relinquishing the stereotyped sex role definition and becoming more androgynous are important for their ego identity as well as care-based moral development.

REFERENCES

Alfieri T, Ruble D, Higgins E. Gender stereotypes during adolescence: Developmental changes and the transition to junior high school. *Developmental Psychology* 1996; 32: 1129-1137.

American Psychiatric association. Practice guideline for the treatment of patients with eating disorders (Revision). *Am J Psychiatry* 2000; 157 (Suppl 1): 1-39.

Andersen A, Holman J. Males with eating disorders: Challenges for treatment and research. *Psychopharmacol Bull* 1997; 33 (3): 391-397.

Andersen A. Gender-related aspects of eating disorders: A guide to practice. *The Journal of Gender-Specific Medicine* 1999; 2(1): 47-54.

Arkkelin D, O'Connor R. The "good" professional: Effect of sex profile gender type, androgyny, and likableness on impressions of incumbents of sex typed occupations. *Sex Roles* 1992; 27 (9-10): 517-532.

Attie I, Brooks-Gunn J. Development of eating problems in adolescent girls: A longitudinal study. *Developmental Psychology* 1989; 25: 70-79.

Basow S. Gender stereotypes and roles. California: Brooks/Cole, 1992.

Behar R. Gender roles and anorexia nervosa. *Acta Psiquiát Psicol Am Lat* 1992; 38 (2): 119-22.

Behar R, De la Barrera M, Michelotti J. Gender identity and eating disorders. *Rev Méd Chile* 2001; 129: 1003-1011.

Behar R, De la Barrera M, Michelotti J. Gender differences in attitudes towards eating behaviors. *Rev Méd Chile* 2002; 130: 964-975.

Behar R, De la Barrera M, Michelotti J. Clinical features and gender identity among eating disordered patient's subtypes. *Rev Méd Chile* 2003; 131: 748-758.

Bem S. The measurement of psychological androgyny. Journal of *Consulting and Clinical psychology* 1974; 42: 155-162.

Bem S. On the utility of alternative procedures for assessing psychological androgyny. *Journal of Consulting and Clinical Psychology* 1977; 45: 196-205.

Bemporad J. Cultural and historical aspects of eating disorders. *Theor Med* 1997; 18: 401-420.

Beren S, Chrisler J. Gender role, need for approval, childness, and self-esteem: markers of disordered eating? *Research Communications in Psychology, Psychiatry and Behavior* 1990; 15(4): 183-198.

Bordo S. *Unbearable weight: Feminism, Western culture, and the body.* Berkeley: University of California Press, 1993.

Boskind-Lodahl M. Cinderella's stepsisters: A feminist perspective on anorexia nervosa and bulimia. *Journal of Women in Culture and Society* 1976; 2: 342-355.

Boskind-Lodahl M, Sirlin J, White WC. The definition and treatment of bulimarexia in college women: A pilot study. *Journal of the American College Health Association* 1978; 27: 84-86.

Boskind-White M, White W. *Bulimarexia: The binge/ purge cycle.* New York: WW Norton, 1983.

Boskind-White M. Bulimarexia: A sociocultural perspective. In: Emmett S, editor. *Theory and treatment of anorexia nervosa and bulimia: Biomedical, sociocultural, and psychological perspectives*. New York: Brunner/Mazel, 1985. p. 113-26.

Bradley J. Autonomy through androgyny. *Nurs Manage* 1993; 24 (10): 64J, 64N-64.

Broverman I et al. Sex role stereotypes: A current appraisal. *Journal of Social Issues* 1972; 28: 59-78.

Brown J, Cross H, Nelson J. Sex role identity and sex role ideology in college women with bulimic behaviour. *Int J Eat Disord* 1990; 9 (5): 571-575.

Brown L, Gilligan C. *Meeting at the crossroads: Women's psychology and girls' development.* New York: Ballantine Books, 1992.

Bruch H. *The golden cage: The enigma of anorexia nervosa*. Cambridge MA: Harvard University Press, 1978.

Brumberg J. *Fasting girls. The emergence of anorexia nervosa as a modern disease.* Cambridge: Harvard University Press, 1988.

Burchardt C, Serbin L. Psychological androgyny and personality adjustment in college and psychiatric populations. *Sex Roles* 1982; 8(8): 835-851.

Cantrell P, Ellis J. Gender role and risk patterns for eating disorders in men and women. *J Clin Psychol* 1991; 47(1): 53-7.

Cauwels J. *Bulimia: The binge-purge compulsion*. New York: Doubleday, 1983.

Crawford C. Effects of sex and sex roles on avoidance of same and opposite sex touch. *Percept Mot Skills* 1994; 79 (1 Pt 1): 107-112.

Crisp A. Anorexia Nervosa. *Hospital Medicine* 1967; 1: 713-718.

Crisp A. Differential diagnosis of anorexia nervosa. *Proc R Soc Med* 1977; 70:686-690.

Crisp A. *Anorexia nervosa. Let me be*. London: Academic Press, 1980.

Chernin K. *The hungry self.* New York: Harper and Row, 1985.

Davis C, Dianne M, Lazarus L. Gender-role orientation and body image in women and men: The moderating influence of neuroticism. *Sex Roles* 1996; 34: 493-505.

Dean C, Gilroy F. Relation of sex-role orientation to life satisfaction in a healthy elderly sample. *Journal of Social Behavior and Personality* 1993; 8(1): 133-140.

Deux K, Major B. Putting gender into context: An interactive model of gender related behaviour. *Psychological Review* 1987; 94: 369-389.

Drewnowski A, Yee D. Men and body image: Are males satisfied with their body weight? *Psychosomatic Medicine* 1987; 49: 626-634.

Emmett S. Future trends. In: Emmett S, editor. *Theory and treatment of anorexia nervosa and bulimia: Biomedical, sociocultural and psychological perspectives.* New York: Brunnel/Mazel, 1985.p. 73-94.

Fallon A, Rozin P. Sex differences in the perception of body shape. *J Abnorm Psychol* 1985; 94: 102-5.

Fornari V, Dancyger IF. Psychosexual development and eating disorders. *Adolesc Med* 2003;14(1):61-75.

Freedman R. *Beauty bound.* Lexington MA: Lexington Books, 1986.

Freedman R. *Body Image: Learning to like our looks and ourselves.* New York: Harper and Row, 1988.

Garfinkel P, Garner D. *Anorexia nervosa: A multidimensional perspective.* New York: Brunner/Mazel, 1982.

Garner D, Garfinkel P, Schwartz D, Thompson M. Cultural expectation of thinness in women. *Psychological Reports* 1980; 47: 483-491.

Garner D, Olmstead M, Bohr I, Garfinfel P. The eating attitudes test: Psychometric features and clinical correlates. *Psychological Med* 1982; 12: 671-8.

Garner D, Garkinfel P, Olmsted M. An overview of sociocultural factors in the development of anorexia nervosa. In: Darby P and others, editors. *Anorexia nervosa: Recent developments in research.* New York: AR Liss. 1983. p. 65-82.

Garner D, Olmstead M, Polivy J. Development and validation of a multidimensional eating disorder inventory for anorexia nervosa and bulimia. *Int J Eat Disord* 1983; 2: 151-34.

Garner D, Rockert W, Johnson C. Psychoeducational principles of bulimia and anorexia nervosa. In: Garner D, Garfinkel P, editors. *Handbook of psychotherapy for anorexia nervosa and bulimia.* New York: Guilford Press, 1985. p. 513-72.

Gilbert S. *Pathology of eating. Psychology and treatment. Social and psychological aspects of medical practice.* London and New York: Routledge and Kegan Paul, 1986.

Gilligan C. *In a different voice: Psychological theory and women's development.* Cambridge: Harvard University Press, 1982.

Greenspan M. *A New Approach to women and therapy.* New York: McGraw-Hill, 1983.

Herman C, Polivy J. Restrained eating. In: Stunkard A, editor. *Obesity.* Philadelphia: Saunders, 1980. p. 208-225.

Herzog D, Bradburn I, Newman K. Sexuality in males with eating disorders. In: Andersen A, editor. *Males with eating disorders.* New York: Brunner/Mazel, 1990. p. 40-53.

Holleran P, Pascale J, Fraley J. Personality correlates of college age bulimics. *Journal of Counselling and Development* 1988; 66: 378-381.

Hawkins R, Clement P. Binge eating syndrome: The measurement problem and a conceptual model. In: Hawkins R, Fremouw W, Clement P, editors. *Binge-eating: Theory, research and treatment.* New York: Springer, 1984. p. 229-251.

Henning K, Strauss B. Personal child-related motives and attitudes in females with eating disorders--indicators for gender role conflicts? *Psychother Psychosom Med Psychol* 2003; 53(1):23-8.

Hsu L. *Eating disorders.* New York: Guilford Press, 1990.

Johnson M. Sex role orientation and attitudes toward sexual expression. *Psychological Reports* 1989; 64(3, Pt 2): 1064.

Johnson M, Brems C, Fischer P. Sex role conflict, social desirability, and eating disorder attitudes and behaviors. *The Journal of General Psychology* 1996; 123: 75-87.

Jones D, Bloys N, Wood M. Sex roles and friendship patterns. *Sex Roles* 1990; 23 (3-4): 133-45.

Katzman MA, Wolchick SA. Bulimia and binge eating in college women: A comparison of personality and behavioral characteristics. *Journal of Consulting and Clinical Psychology* 1984; 52: 428-523.

Kearney-Cooke A. Gender differences and self-esteem. *J Gend Specif Med* 1999; 2(3):46-52.

Klingenspor B. Gender identity and bulimic eating behavior. *Sex Roles* 1994; 31: 407-431.

Kohlberg L. A cognitive developmental analysis of children's sex role concepts and attitudes. In: Maccoby E, editor. *The development of sex differences.* Stanford: Stanford University Press, 1966. p. 82-193

Lancelot C, Kaslow J. Sex role orientation and disordered eating in women: A review. *Clinical Psychology Review* 1994; 14 (2): 139-157.

Levine M. *How schools can help combat student eating disorders: Anorexia nervosa and bulimia*. Washington DC: National Education Association, 1987.

Lewinsohn P, Mischel W, Chaplin W, Barton R. Social competence and depression: The role of illusory self-perceptions. *J of Abnormal Psychol* 1980; 89: 203-12.

Lewis L, Johnson C. A comparison of sex role orientation between women with bulimia and normal controls. *Int J Eat Disord* 1985; 4: 247-257.

Mead B, Ignico A. Children's gender typed perceptions of physical activity: Consequences and implications. *Percept Mot Skills* 1992; 75: (3 Pt 2): 1035-42.

Meyer C, Blissett J, Oldfield C. Sexual orientation and eating psychopathology: The role of masculinity and femininity. *Int J Eat Disord* 2001; 29(3):314-8.

Miller M, Pumariega A. Culture and eating disorders: A historical and cross-cultural review. *Psychiatry* 2001; 64 (2): 93-110.

Mintz L, Betz N. Sex differences in the nature, realism, and correlates of body image. *Sex Roles* 1986; 15: 185-195.

Morawski J. The measurement of masculinity and femininity: Engendering categorical realities. In: Bohan J, editor. *Seldom seen, rarely heard: Woman's place in psychology*. Boulder: Westview Press, 1992. p. 199-226.

Murnen S, Smolak L. Femininity, masculinity, and disordered eating: A meta-analytic review. *Int J Eat Disord* 1997; 22: 231-242.

Napholz L. Indices if psychological well-being and sex role orientation among working women. *Health Care Women Int* 1994; 15 (4): 307-16.

Nassar M. Eating disorders: The cultural dimension. *Soc Psychiatry Psychiatr Epidemiol* 1988; 23: 184-187.

Orbach S. *Fat is a feminine issue. The anti-diet guide to permanent weight loss.* New York: Paddington Press, 1978.

Orbach S. Visibility/Invisibility: Social considerations in anorexia nervosa (A feminist perspective. In: Emmett S, editor. *Theory and treatment of anorexia nervosa and bulimia: Biomedical, sociocultural, and psychological perspectives*. New York: Brunner/Mazel, 1985. p. 127-38.

Orbach S. *Hunger strike. The anorectic's struggle as a metaphor for our age*. New York: Faber and Faber, 1986.

Orlofsky J. Psychological androgyny, sex-typing, and sex-role ideology as predictors of male-female interpersonal attraction. *Sex Roles* 1982; 8: 1057 - 1073.

Palazzoli M. *Self-starvation. From individual to family therapy in the treatment of anorexia nervosa*. New York: Jason Aronson, 1978.

Paxton S, Sculthorpe A. Disordered eating and sex role characteristics in young women: Implications for sociocultural theories of disturbed eating. *Sex Roles* 1991; 24: 587-598.

Pliner P, Chaiken S, Flett G. Gender differences in concern with body weight and physical appearance over the life span. *Personality and Social Psychology Bulletin* 1990; 16: 263-273.

Polivy J, Herman P. *Breaking the diet habit*. New York: Basic Books, 1983.

Polivy J, Garner D, Garfinkel P. Causes and consequences of the current preference for thin female physics. In: Herman C, Zanna M, Higgins E, editors. *Physical appearance, stigma, and social behavior: The third Ontario symposium in personality and social psychology*. New Jersey: Erlbaum, 1986. p. 89-112.

Pope K, Hudson J. Anorexia nervosa and "reverse anorexia" among 108 male bodybuilders. *Compr Psychiatry* 1993; 34 (6): 406-409.

Prince R. The concept of culture-bound-syndromes: Anorexia nervosa and brain-fag. *Soc Sc Med* 1985; 21: 197-203.

Pursell S, Banikiotes P, Sebastian R. Androgyny and the perception of marital roles. *Sex Roles* 1981; 7: 201-215.

Rewal V, Kapur V. Sex roles: Masculinity, femininity and androgyny as a function of age, sex and city. *Journal of Personality and Clinical Studies* 1991; 7(1): 67-72.

Ricards L, McAlister L. Female submissiveness, nonverbal behavior, and body boundary definition. *J Psychol* 1994; 128 (4): 419-24.

Rodin J, Silberstein L, Striegel-Moore R. Women and weight: A normative discontent. In: Sonderegger T, editor. *Nebraska Symposium on Motivation, 1984: Psychology and gender*. Lincoln: University of Nebraska, 1985. p. 267-308.

Root P. Disordered eating in women of color. *Sex Roles* 1990; 22: 525-536.

Rost H, Neuhaus M, Florin O. Bulimia nervosa: Sex role attitudes, sex role behavior, and sex role related locus of control in bulimarexic women. *Journal of Psychosomatic Research* 1982; 26: 240-244.

Schwartz D, Thompson M, Johnson C. Eating disorders and the culture. In: Anorexia nervosa and bulimia: The sociocultural context. *Int J Eat Disord* 1982; 1: 20-36.

Siever M. Sexual orientation and gender as factors in socioculturally acquired vulnerability to body dissatisfaction and eating disorders. *J Consult Clin Psychol* 1994; 62(2): 252-60.

Silverstein B, Perdue L, Wolf C, Pizzolo C. Binging, purging, and estimates of parental attitudes regarding female achievement. *Sex Roles* 1988; 19: 723-733.

Silverstein B, Carpman S, Perlick D, Perdue L. Nontraditional sex role aspirations, gender identity conflict, and disordered eating among college women. *Sex Roles* 1990; 23: 687-695.

Silverstein B, Perlick D. *The cost of competence: Why inequality causes depression, eating disorders, and illness in women*. New York: Oxford University Press, 1995.

Singleton C. Biological and social explanations of sex-role stereotyping. In: Hargreaves D, Colley A, editors. *The Psychology of sex roles*. Cambridge: Hemisphere, 1987. p. 3-26.

Shimonaka Y, Nakazato K, Marushima R. Androgyny and psychological well-being among older and younger Japanese adults. *Aging Milano* 1994; 6(1): 43-8.

Shimonaka Y, Nakazato K, Kawaai C, Sato S. Androgyny and successful adaptation across the life span among Japanese adults. *J Genet Psychol* 1997; 158 (4): 389-400.

Skoe E. Sex role orientation and its relationship to the development of identity and moral thought. *Scand J Psychol* 1995; 36 (3): 235-45.

Slade R. *The anorexia nervosa reference book*. London: Harper and Row, Publishers, 1984.

Smolak L, Levine M. Toward an empirical basis for primary prevention of eating problems with elementary school children. Eating disorders: *Journal of Treatment and prevention* 1994; 4: 293-307.

Spence J, Helmreich R, Stapp J. Ratings of self and peers on sex roles attributes and their relations to self-esteem and conceptions of masculinity and femininity. *Journal of Personality and Social Psychology* 1975; 32: 29-39.

Spence J, Helmreich R. *Masculinity and femininity: Their psychological dimensions, correlates and antecedents*. Austin: University of Texas Press, 1978.

Steenbarger B, Greenberg R. Sex roles, stress, and distress: A study of person by situation contingency. *Sex Roles* 1990; 22(1-2): 59-68.

Steiner-Adair C. The body politic: Normal female adolescent development and the development of eating disorders. *Journal of the American Academy of Psychoanalysis* 1986; 14: 95-114.

Steiner-Adair C. Developing the voice of the wise woman: College students and bulimia. *Journal of College Student Psychotherapy* 1989; 3: 151-165.

Stice E. Review of the evidence for a sociocultural model of bulimia nervosa and an exploration of the mechanisms of action. *Clinical Psychology Review* 1994; 14(7): 633-661.

Stice E, Schupak E, Shaw H, Stein R. Relation of media exposure to eating disorder symptomatology: An examination of mediating mechanisms. *J Abnorm Psychol* 1994; 103 (4): 836-40.

Striegel-Moore R, Silberstein L, Rodin J. Towards an understanding of risk factors for bulimia. *American Psychologist* 1986; 41: 246-63.

Swarr A, Richards M. Longitudinal Effects of Adolescent Girls. Pubertal Development, Perceptions of Pubertal Timing, and Parental Relations on Eating Problems. *Developmental Psychology* 1996; 32: 636-646.

Szymanski L, Chrisler J. Eating disorders, gender role and athletic activity. Special issue: Special Recognition to Dr. Russell N. Cassel. *Psychology a Journal of Human Behaviour* 1990-91; 27 (4) – 28 (1): 20-29.

Thomä H. *Anorexia nervosa*. New York: International University Press, 1967.

Thomas K, Ricciardelli L. Gender traits and self-concept: Indicators of problem eating and body dissatisfaction among children. *Sex Roles* 2000;

Thornton B, Leo R, Alberg K. Gender role typing, the superwoman ideal, and the potential for eating disorders. *Sex Roles* 1991; 25: 469-484.

Troop NA, Allan S, Treasure JL, Katzman M. Social comparison and submissive behaviour in eating disorder patients. *Psychol Psychother* 2003; 76(Pt 3):237-49.

Usmiani S, Daniluk J. Mothers and their adolescent daughters: Relationship between self-esteem, gender role identity and body image. *Journal of Youth and Adolescence* 1997; 26(1), 45-61.

Vandereycken W, Hoek H. Are eating disorders culture-bound syndrome? In: Halmi K, editor. *Psychobiology and treatment of anorexia nervosa and bulimia nervosa*. Washington DC: American Psychiatric Association, 1992. p. 19-38.

Vonk R, Ashmore R. The multifaceted self: Androgyny reassessed by open ended self descriptions. *Social Psychology Quarterly* 1993; 56(4): 278-287.

Wooley S, Wooley O. Intensive outpatient and residential treatment for bulimia. In: Garner D, Garfinkel P, editors. *Handbook of psychotherapy for anorexia nervosa and bulimia.* New York: Guilford Press, 1985. p. 391-430.

Wooley S. Sexual abuse and eating disorders: The concealed debate. In: Fallon P, Katzman M, Wooley S, editors. *Feminine perspectives on eating disorders.* New York: Guilford Press, 1994. p. 171.211.

Yarnold P, Martin G, Soltysik R, Nightingale S. Androgyny predicts empathy for trainees in medicine. *Percept Mot Skills* 1993; 77(2): 576-8.

In: Eating Disorders and Weight Loss Research
Editor: Jerome S. Rubin, pp. 67-76
ISBN 1-60021-334-0

Chapter 3

BULIMIC BEHAVIOR IN ADOLESCENT ATHLETES

Maria Lúcia Bosi[1] and Fátima Palha de Oliveira
Federal University of Rio de Janeiro - Brasil

ABSTRACT

Introduction

Eating disorders are today an increasing problem among teenagers and young adults specially females. In the case of bulimia the estimated prevalence is between 3 and 5% and the average age it starts is around 20 years. It is known that its etiology is complex and depends on biological, psychological, and social factors as well as more specific characteristics as, for example, the practice of sports that in some cases leads to these disorders. The close relation between corporal image and performance makes the female athletes a group particularly vulnerable to problems of bulimic behavior due to the emphasis in weight control that they are frequently submitted. However the studies available are still insufficient to characterize the amplitude and distribution of the problem.

Objective

The aim of the present work is to evaluate bulimic components of behavior among adolescent female endurance runners.

Methods

From a total of 40 athletes affiliated with the Track and Field Federation of Rio de Janeiro, 17 female endurance runners (16 ± 1.8 years old) and 32 post-menarche, non-athletic adolescents (15.0 ± 1.4 years) were examined. The athletes were training for at least 2 years (15 ± 7 hours/week).

---

[1] Address for correspondence: Rua Octávio de Rezende, 1060/600 Meireles - Fortaleza Ceará – Brazil email: ***malubosi@nesc.ufrj.br***

The body composition was esteemed by the anthropometric method and percent body fat (%F) and Body Mass Index (BMI) were calculated. Bulimic behavioral components (frequency and severity) were evaluated using the Portuguese version of BITE (Bulimic Investigatory Test, Edinburgh), a self-rating scale.

A control group of 32 non-athlete volunteers in the same age group were also evaluated. Calculation of parameters, descriptive data statistics and comparison (Anova one way) of the variables were performed with the software Statistica for windows (5.1, 1998), with a significant level of $p \leq 0,05$.

Results and Discussion

Scores above the normal limit of 10 were recorded for 35.3% of the athletes (6 individuals), including 29.4% (4 individuals) that reported unusual behavioral components, suggestive of a tendency toward bulimia. One individual scored above 20, indicating a possible clinical case of bulimia. On the scale of severity of the symptoms, a score of 5 (considered moderately severe) was recorded in one case.

Conclusions

The athletes in this group are in risk to develop eating disorder, considering their preoccupation with weight control and the use of inadequate means of keeping within the desired range – including restrictive practices such as fasting along with intense physical activity.

Keywords: Bulimia, Eating Disorders, Athletes.

INTRODUCTION

Eating disorders are defined as deviations in eating behavior that correspond essentially to anorexia nervosa and bulimia nervosa. Depending on the classification used, non-specific eating disorders may also be included, such as compulsive or binge eating[1].

A number of authors [2-5] have pointed out that anorexia and bulimia appear to be on the rise in recent years, affecting in particular young (adolescent) women, a population that is at the highest risk for these disorders. Both bulimic and anorexic behaviors are resistant to treatment, and anorexia nervosa can be lethal in 5% to 20% of the cases in which it occurs[3]. Individuals with these disorders have in common an excessive preoccupation with weight and diet, as well as self-dissatisfaction and a distorted self-image.

In addition, the disorder referred to as compulsive periodic eating – a syndrome included in Appendix B of the DSM-IV[6] – must be considered a serious problem in the population as a whole[7,8] since it is closely correlated with obesity, a condition that is widely recognized as a public health problem among adults in Brazil [9-13].

Bulimia nervosa, the primary focus in this study, is estimated to affect between 3% and 5% of adolescents and young adults in the female population[14.]

This syndrome is characterized by repeated bouts of overeating and an excessive preoccupation with the control of body weight, leading the patient to adopt extreme measures so as to mitigate the 'fattening" effects of ingested food.

Individuals with bulimia consume large quantities of food, especially when subjected to stressful situations, and subsequently develop compensatory behaviors in order to avoid gaining weight and to alleviate the sense of guilt and shame evoked by uncontrolled eating[15].

Because of the "secret" character of this ritual, bulimia is difficult to diagnose, especially in its initial phase, and is therefore difficult to prevent as well as to treat at an early stage.

Although the prevalence of bulimia among female athletes in Brazil has not been adequately documented, reports from other countries indicate a higher frequency than among non-athletes, especially in certain sports[18] that emphasize leanness for performance and appearance the athletes. Thus, gymnasts, long-distance runners, dancers, and figure skaters are more prone to developing eating disorders and related problems than those who compete in nonweight-restricting sports such as volleyball or football [18]. The prevalence of eating disorders is higher among female athletes than nonathletes[19,20] and the estimates of eating disorders among athletes range between 15% to 62%[21]. Sundegot-Borge[21] observed a hight prevalence of eating disorders and the inadequate weight control was significantly higher among bodybuilders (34%) and those who practice sports tha require low body mass (27%). For technical (13%) or team sports (11%), the prevalence was lower, and the control present a prevalence of 7%.

The close relationship between corporal image and physical performance makes female athletes especially vulnerable to the development of bulimic behaviors and other eating disorders, in view of the emphasis given to weight control as part of the training regime. Rosen and Hough (apud Ruud, 1996) point to the influence exerted by coach' comments about athletes' weight and form as an important factor in promoting adoption of abnormal eating behaviors. In addition, the prescription of restrictive diets at an early age, especially in the absence of professional supervision, can lead to serious damage to an athlete's health and consequently to her athletic performance. The reduce plasma volume impaired thermoregulation and nutrient exchange, decreased glycogen availability and decrease buffer capacity in the blood are a possible explanation for reduced performance, especially after rapid weith reduction[22].

Inadequate nutrition can cause in female athletes, whose energy requirements are different from those of non-athletic women, problems such as amenorrhea, loss of bone density, anemia, and behavioral anomalies such as bulimia and/or anorexia. Inadequate eating habits can give rise to mineral depletion and osteoporosis, making bones more fragile. Osteoporosis is one component of the so-called *women athletes' triad* (amenorrhea, eating disorder, and osteoporosis) that results from dietary intake that is unequal to the athlete's daily energy demand. The literature indicates that 90% of those who suffer from osteoporosis are women[23], a statistic that coincides with the distribution of bulimia and other eating disorders.

Eating disorders constitute not only a significant clinical picture among individuals, but also an increasingly troublesome question of public health[1]. Statistics for Latin America show that in the last 10 years there has been a nearly exponential increase in eating disorders, leading to coefficients of prevalence and incidence greater than those in the United States.

In Brazil, it has been estimated that about 19% of female students exhibit symptoms of bulimia[26] – that is, behavior that can be taken to indicate that a full-blown clinical manifestation of bulimia nervosa is imminent. In addition, in one of the few population studies available, a survey in Pelotas (in the state of Rio Grande do Sul) showed a prevalence of 13.8% in the practice of anomalous eating behaviors, indicating subclinical development of the classical syndromes, while 30.2% exhibited behavior characteristic of individuals at risk and 11.3% clearly showed abnormal eating behavior that could be classified among the non-specific eating disorders[3].

Nevertheless, there are clearly recognizable precursor stages of these disorders, and they are much more prevalent than the fully developed clinical disorders[1]. From the point of view of prevention, it is essential to be able to recognize these early signs. This implies cooperative interaction between the investigative teams and family members.

Among the identified subclinical syndromes are the use of restrictive diets, the practice of self-induced vomiting, and the use of laxatives, diuretics and/or anorexogenic drugs, associated with strenuous physical activity. Any of these signs can serve as a warning to take action against further development of the clinical disorders.

These considerations define a context in which research on this topic can be expected to provide feedback that will be useful to the services, the teaching and the training of future investigators on this topic. The objective of the present study is to help define the dimensions of the problem in one of its specific manifestations – bulimia and its behavioral precursors – within a population that is at risk: female adolescent athletes in training for a specific event. We present it as a first step in an already expanding effort to include other sports and population groups, in the expectation of contributing to the definition and comprehension of a complex theme that involves bio-psychic, epidemiologic, anthropologic, sociologic economic and historical aspects [27-32] – and therefore one that requires an interdisciplinary approach capable of integrating these different facets.

Material and Method

A transverse study design was employed, using subjects from a population that is considered to be at greatest risk for the development of eating disorders: adolescent females, especially athletes[33, 34].

The sample consisted of 17 adolescents (15.9 ± 1.8 years) chosen at random from a population of 40 adolescent athletes who were registered at the time in the *Track and Field Federation of Rio de Janeiro*. The athletes were training for at least 2 years (15 ± 7 hours/week). Criteria for including these individuals in the study were as follows:

- All 17 athletes had been engaged in a systematic training program under supervision of a professional trainer, in different athletic clubs in Rio de Janeiro, for at least two years, on an average of 15 hours per week.
- All were training for endurance events of 800 m or more.
- All of the individuals chosen had been classified above fifth place in a recent juvenile competition in the state of Rio de Janeiro.

Also evaluated was a control group of volunteers consisting of 32 post-menarche, non-athletic adolescents aged 15.0 ± 1.4 years.

In order to evaluate the presence and intensity of bulimic behaviors, the Bulimic Investigatory Test of Edinburgh (BITE)[26, 35] was used. This is a self-administered questionnaire consisting of 33 questions, with two subscales – one related to the symptoms and one to the severity of the symptoms. The scale for symptoms is subdivided into High (20 points or more), Medium (10 to 19 points) and Low (below 10 points). The scale for severity of symptoms is subdivided into Light (score below 5), Moderate (5 to 9) and Severe (greater than 10), and is used in those cases where the score in the first scale (symptoms) is greater than 10. In the present study, the Portuguese version was used [26.] Results were tabulated according to frequency (absolute and relative values).

To obtain a profile of the athletes' body composition he follow anthropometrical measurements were taken:

Skinfolds thikness (mm:) The mean of three skinfold measurements were registraded for the following points: triceps, medium axilla, subscapula, suprailiac, abdomen, biceps, thigh, and leg, using a Cescorf compass with a precision of 0.1 mm.

Body weight (kg, precision of 50 g) and *height* (m, precision of 1 mm) — in lightbclothing and without shoes — were measured using calibrates scales.

From the measures fond, the parameters were calculated:

The *percentage of body fat* (%F)[36]was obtained from *body density* estimated according to the equation developed by Withers et al. (1987)[37] specifically for female athletes. The *percentage of* body fat in the control group was calculated as described by Jackson et al.(1980)[38].

The *Body Mass Index* was calculated as the ratio of weight (kg) to h eight (m^2) (BMI= weight / Heigth^2)[39.]

The anthropometric readings are reported as average and standard deviation for the group. Calculation of parameters, descriptive data statistics and comparison (t Student) of the variables were performed with the softwere "Statistica for windows" (6.0, 2001). The statistical significance level adopted in these analyses was 5% ($p \leq 0.05$).

This study was carried out with the written consent of the participants, who were also informed about the planned use of the data obtained.

Results and Discussion

The characteristics of the subjects' body composition are shown in Table 1.

Athletes had weight, body fat and body mass index significantly lower than the control group, but there are no significant difference for age and height.

This result is to be expected for endurance runners, whose training is directed toward increasing their aerobic resistance. One of the adaptive responses to this training is a greater reliance on lipids as a source of energy. This adaptation has a pronounced impact on body composition of female athletes who run long distances, and they tend to have less body fat than athletes in other sports[23].

Studies have found that , even with body mass within normal populations standarts,it is significant the numbers of yong women unhappy with their weight and that do inappropriate practices to reduces body mass[24]. The young athletes had a aditional pressure concern body size and shape by the social influence for thinness, anxiety about athletic performance and negative self-appraisal of athletic achievement[25].

Table 1. Anthropometric Characteristics

Group	Age (years)	Weight (Kg)	Height (cm)	Body fat (%)	BMI (Kg/m2)
Athletes (17)	15.9 ± 1.8	49.3 ± 5.2	161.9 ± 5.6	22.0 4.2	18.8 ± 1.9
Controls (32)	15.0 ± 1.4	58.0 ± 11.0	162.5 ± 6.5	26.5 ± 8.1	22.0 ± 4.0
T Student (p)		0.004*		0.044*	0.004*

BMI= Body Mass Index; * signifficant difference p ≤ 0,05.

Our investigation confirm this possibility when observed that in spite of the normal ranges[23] encountered for body mass, body fat and body mass index among the athletes, the results of the BITE questionnaire indicated the presence of pre-bulimic behaviors and even, in one case, a possibility of bulimia.

Results of the BITE

Analysis of the athletes' answers to the BITE (Table 2) indicated that 35.3% (n=6) had scores above 10, the limit of the normal range. Of this percentage, 29.4% responded with an anomalous pattern (scores of 10 – 19), indicating behavior suggestive of a risk of bulimia. A value above 19 identified one individual (5.9% of the total) as a strong possibility of having fully developed bulimia. In the control group, a smaller proportion (21.8%) had scores in the 10 to 19 range, i.e. above the normal limit. The result is in accord of Sundegot-Borgen`[21] thatobserved a higth prevalence of eating disorders in athletes (18%) than in no-athletes (5%).

On the scale for severity one athlete had score greater than 10 (severe) and the others (n=5) achieved scores below 5 (light).

Table 2. Result of the Bite

	ATHLETES	CONTROL
Synptom Scale		
HIGH (> 20 points)	5,9 %	0%
MÉDIUM (10 – 19 points)	29,4 %	21,8%
LOW (or within normal range) (below 10 points)	64,7 %	78,2%
Severity Scale Applied when changes in the synptom scale were found		
SEVERE (greater than 10)	16,6 %	0%
MODERATE (5 to 9 points): clinically signifficant	0%	9,4 %
LIGHT (score below 5 points): clinically *non* signifficant	83,3 %	87,5%

Table 3 presents some of BITE questions were one can see the concern with weigth control and practice of dietary restrictions, particulary fasting, which are conflicting with physical activities.

Table 3. Among The Findings, A Number of Replies Suggested Bulimic Behavior

Behavioral characteristic	**Prevalence in athletes**	**Prevalence in controls**
1 – Fear (horror) of getting fat; eating large quantities of food very rapidly	58.8%	46.8%
2 – Fasting for an entire day	*52.9%*	*18.7%*
3 – Accustomed to eating when not observed	*52.9%*	*31.2%*
4 – Worried about lack of control over eating	47.1%	53.1%
5 – Feeling of guilt when eating	41.2%	53.1%
6 – Obsessive thoughts about food	29.4%	*31.2%*

Questions from BITE, portraing dietary practice and emitional attiitude

The result of revealed the abnormal eating behaviors in athlete and control groups, that reflect a possible subclinical eating disorder syndromes[40]. The subclinical cases have a higth prevalence among athletes[41] and the early identification and intervention in these groups may prevent development of the eating disorder[42].

Less frequently, other types of behavior were also mentioned by the athletes, including a tendency to eat more when anxious (17.6%); fluctuations in weight (23.5%); and feelings of shame about food and one's own eating habits (17.6%).

Oliveira *et al.* [43] show in athletes of differents sports modalities the presence of worriment about body weigh, combined with a mild distortion of body image and also the practice of dietary restriction. The authors alerted to such parcial eating disorder syndromes associed to systematic and exhaustible physical exercise is a risk factors of eating disorders.

From the data of these study, it is apparent that the athletic individuals in this group are in risk to develop bulimia, especially considering their preoccupation with weight control and the use of inadequate means of keeping within the desired range – including restrictive practices such as fasting along with intense physical activity (table 2).

In addition to the risk of these young athletes' developing eating disorders, it is disturbing to find these signs of abnormal eating behavior in a group that is undergoing rapid physical development and is under training. A systematic training program generates a daily energy demand that requires adequate attention to nutrition. A long-term low energyy intake may impede the athlete from reaching her full potential and, moreover, lead to a negative consequences, such as inadequate carbohydrate, protein, vitamin and mineral intake, increased risk of injury and increased risk of illness [44].

At the other extreme, the loss of control over food intake is an element that stands out, along with feelings associated with these practices – guilt, shame, fear, anxiety – a whole gamut of emotions that are characteristic of bulimia and represent a psychic suffering that should not be neglected, not only because of the emotional vulnerability of this age group but also because of the pressure associated with performing well in a highly competitive milieu. It is relevant to consider the possibly synergistic effects of these emotional factors in contributing to the development of eating disorders as well as to the difficulty in managing them.

Conclusion

As we have tried to show, eating disorders, including bulimia, represent a disturbing problem that appears to be increasing, especially among adolescent females and young women. With regard to female athletes, nutritional planning should focus on bulimia as a possible complication of the close relationship between diet and training for sports, considering the daily demands with regard to weight and form, as well as the stress of competition.

In fact, it is no surprise that in the self-administered test included in the present report there appear multiple behavioral signs pointing toward individuals at risk of developing bulimia, or even with clinically apparent bulimia, still in a comparatively mild form.

Professionals who deal with this segment of the population – MD's, physical education teachers, psychologists and nutritionists, among other specialists – need to be well informed and trained to identify and manage bulimia. Detecting signs of this disorder and intervening at an early stage are essential in order to preserve not only an athlete's performance but also her health, recognizing that a healthy diet and mental stability are fundamental to physical activity.

In the future, further studies should be aimed at evaluating the dimensions of the problem in this and other groups at risk, as well as broadening the field of inquiry to include a qualitative description of the genesis of these behaviors -- still an engima in many aspects.

Acknowledgment

We thank Professor Marta Sorenson for revision of the article and the staff of the LABOFISE. This study was parcially funded by FAPERJ AND FUJB.

A preliminary version of this study were publicated as short comunication in Brasilian Journal of Psychiatry, 2004, 26(1):32-34.

References

[1] American Psychiatric Association. Diagnostic and Statistical Manual of Mental Disorders, 4th Ed. Washington: American Psychiatric Association; 1994.

[2] Russell, G. Bulimia Nervosa: an ominous variant of anorexia nervosa. *Psychol. Medicine*, 1979, 9:429-48.

[3] Nunes, MAA. Prevalência de Comportamentos Alimentares Anormais e Práticas Inadequadas de Controle de Peso em Mulheres de 12 a 21 anos em Porto Alegre. PortoAlegre, 1997. Dissertação (mestrado). Universidade Federal de Pelotas.

[4] Nunes, MAA . Influência da Percepção do peso e do índice de massa corporal nos comportamentos alimentares anormais. *Revista Brasileira de Psiquiatria,* 2001 23:21-7.

[5] ANDRADE, AC. Para além dos sintomas: a trilogia do desamparo no vivido de mulheres com transtornos do comportamento alimentar. Dissertação de

Mestrado/Universidade Federal do Ceará. Mestrado em saúde Pública/Departamento de saúde Comunitária. 2000.
[6] Manual diagnóstico e estatístico de transtornos mentais DSM-IV. Tradução de Dayse Batista. Porto Alegre: Artes Médicas; 1995.
[7] Appolinário, JC. transtorno do comer compulsivo. In: Abuchaim, ALG, Appolinário, JC; Nunes, MAA; Coutinho, W; *et al.*, editores. Transtornos Alimentares e Obesidade. Porto Alegre: Artes Médicas; 1998; 40-46.
[8] Appolinário, JC. Transtorno da compulsão alimentar periódica e transtorno obssessivo-compulsivo: partes de um mesmo espectro? *Revista Brasileira de Psiquiatria*, 2001 23:38-40.
[9] Hollis, JM. Une affaire de famille. Montreal: Éditions Sciences et Culture; 1992.
[10] Hoek, H. The Distribution of eating disorders. In: Brownell, KD; Fairburn, CG, editores. Eating Disorders and Obesity. A Comprehensive Handbook. New York: The Guilford Press;1995.
[11] Gigante, DP. Prevalência de obesidade em adultos e seus fatores de risco. *Revista de Saúde Pública*, 1997 31:236-46.
[12] Sichieri, R. Epidemiologia da obesidade. Rio de Janeiro: Editora UERJ; 1998.
[13] Jimenéz, R. La percepción de la función familiar y el desarrollo psicosexual en el adolescente obeso. *Revista de Investigación Clinica*, 1992 44:525-30.
[14] Morandé, G; Carrera, M. Anorexias nerviosas y bulimias. Una epidemia actual en adolescentes? Algunos aspectos en discussion. *Revista de Psiquiatria do Chile*, 1988, (1):19-28.
[15] Castilla, D; Bastin, C. La boulimie: mieux se connaître pour en guérir. Paris: Éd. Robert Laffont; 1998.
[16] Maine, M. Anorexie, boulimie, pourquoi? Paris, Barretle-bas: Le souffle d'or, 1997.
[17] Paleo, MC. Anorexia y bulimia nerviosa – comunicacion humana y sistemas humanos. Centro Médico de Mar del Plata, 7, p. 16-19, 1994. Mimeo.
[18] Ruud, JS. Nutrition and the female athlete. New York: CRC Press; 1996.
[19] Sundgot-Borgen, J. Eating disorders in female athletes. *Sports Med*icine 1994 17:176-88.
[20] Yeager, KK; Agostini, R; Nattiv, A; Drinkwater, B. The female athlete triad – disordered eating, amenorrhea and osteoporosis. *Medicine andScience in Sports and Exercise,* 1993 25:775-7.
[21] Sundgot-Borgen, J. Prevalence of eating disorders in elite female athletes. *International Journal of Sport and Nutrition,* 1993 3:29-34.
[22] Fogelholm, M. Effects of the body weight reduction on sports performance. *Sports Medicine,* 1994 4:249-67.
[23] Mcardle, WD; Katch, FI; Katch, VL. Essencials of exercise physiology. second edition. Philadelphia: Lippincott Williams and Wilkins; 2000.
[24] King, MA. Eating disorders in a general practice population: prevalence, characteristics and follow-up at 12 to 18 months. *Physichol Mededicine,* 1989 14:211-18.
[25] Williamson, DA; Netemeyer, RG; Jackman, LP; Anderson, DA; Funsch, CL; Rabalais, JY. Structural equation modeling of risk factors for the development of eating disorder symptoms in female athletes. *International Journal of Eating Disorders,* 1995 17:387-93.

[26] Cordás, TA; Hochgraf, PB. O BITE: Instrumento para avaliação da bulimia nervosa. Versão para o português. *Jornal Brasileiro de Psiquiatria*, 1993 42:141-4.

[27] Bourdieu, P. La domination masculine. Paris: Seuil; 1998.

[28] Leloup, JY. O corpo e seus símbolos: uma antropologia essencial. 3ª edição Petrópolis: Vozes, 1998.

[29] Guillemot, A; Laxenaire, M. Anorexie mentale et boulimie – le poids de la culture. 2e édicion. Paris: Masson; 1997.

[30] Breilh, J. El Genero entrefuegos: inequidad y esperanza. Quito: CEAS; 1996.

[31] Pasini, W. Nourriture and amour. Paris: Payot; 1994.

[32] Balasc, C. Désir de rien. Paris: Aubier; 1990.

[33] Kaplan, HI; Sadock, BJ; Grebb, JA. Compêndio de psiquiatria. 7ª edição. Porto Alegre: Artes Médicas; 1997.

[34] Nunes, MAA; Ramos, DC. Anorexia nervosa: classificação diagnóstica e quadro clínico. In: Nunes, MAA; Coutinho, W; *et al.* Transtornos alimentares e obesidade. Porto Alegre: Artes Médicas; 1998; 21-30.

[35] Henderson, M; Freeman, CPL. A self-rating scale for bulimia. The BITE. *British Journal of Psychiatry,* 1987 50:18-24.

[36] Siri, WE. Gross composition of the body In: Lawrence, J; Tobias, CA. Advanced in biological and medical physics. New York: Academic Press; 1956.

[37] Withers, RT; Whittingham, NO; Norton, KL; Laforgia, J; Ellis, MW; Crockett, A. Relative body fat and anthropometric prediction of body density of female athletes. *European Journal of Applied Physiology*, 1987 56:169-80.

[38] Jackson, AS; Pollock, ML; Ward, A . Generalized equation for predicting body density of women. *Medicine and Science in Sports and Exercise,* 1980 12:175- 82.

[39] Quetelet, A. Antropométrie ou mesure dês différentes facultes de l'homme. Bruxelles: C.Muquardt; 1870.

[40] Nunes, MAA. Prevalência de comportamentos alimentares anormais e práticas inadequadas de controle de peso em mulheres de 12 a 21 anos em Porto Alegre. Porto Alegre [Dissertação de mestrado]. Porto Alegre (RS): Universidade Federal de Pelotas; 1997b.

[41] Grange, D L; Tibbs J, Noakes, T. Implication of a diagnosis of anorexia nervosa in a ballet school. *International Journal of eating disorders,* 1994 4:369-76.

[42] Bassoe, HH. Anorexia/Blimia nervosa: the development of anorexia nervosa and of mental symptom. Tratament and the outcome of the disease Acta *Psychiatrica Scandinavica,* 1990 82:7-13.

[43] Oliveira, FP; Bosi, MLM; Vigário, PS; Vieira, RS. Eating behavior and body image in athletes. *Revista Brsileira de Medicina do Esporte (Brasilian Journal of Sport Medicine),* 2004 9:1-8.

[44] Grandjean, AC; Ruud, JS; Reimers, KJ. Nutrition. In: Women in sport. Drinkwater, BL, editor. Australia: Blackwell Science; 2000; 120-31.

In: Eating Disorders and Weight Loss Research
Editor: Jerome S. Rubin, pp. 77-104
ISBN 1-60021-334-0

Chapter 4

A REVIEW OF BEHAVIORAL INTERVENTIONS TO REDUCE THE RUMINATION OF PERSONS WITH DEVELOPMENTAL DISABILITIES

David B. McAdam and Lynn Cole
University of Rochester

ABSTRACT

Rumination is the regurgitation of recently ingested food and is one of the most commonly occurring eating disorders in persons with developmental disabilities. Rumination might result in the negative side effect of foul breath and can interfere with a person's opportunities to engage in social interactions. Additionally, medical side effects include weight loss, aspiration pneumonia, and tooth decay. The published research studies that examined the efficacy of behavioral-intervention packages to reduce rumination are summarized in this chapter. This chapter also reviews the clinical effectiveness and generality of these intervention packages and highlights recent clinical advancements in the treatment of rumination.

Keywords: rumination; developmental disabilities; behavioral interventions

I. INTRODUCTION

In both typically developing persons and persons with developmental disabilities, rumination is described as the effortless regurgitation of recently ingested food (Chial et al., 2003). A normal process that facilitates complete digestion in some animals such as sheep, cattle, and goats, rumination is not typically displayed by humans, and the behavior is associated with a variety of potential negative side effects (Malcom et al., 1997). Medical complications may include weight loss, aspiration pneumonia, dehydration, electrolyte imbalance, esphagitis, malnutrition, tooth decay, and lowered resistance to disease (Chial et al., 2003, O'Brien, Bruce and Camilleri, 1995, Starin and Fuqua, 1987). In severe cases, rumination can be life-threatening and several authors have described cases in which rumination has contributed to a person's death (Dudley, Johnson, and Barnes, 2002). Persons with developmental disabilities who display rumination often experience the additional negative-side effect of fetid breath and foul odor from contact between vomitus and the person's body and clothing. Rumination may interfere with an individual's opportunities to engage in social interactions by increasing the probability that other people will avoid them in social situations. In addition, rumination may result in significant school and work absenteeism, hospitalizations, and medical attention resulting in compromised daily functioning (Chial et al, 2003).

The purpose of this chapter is to review the published literature on behavioral interventions to reduce rumination of persons with developmental disabilities. Additionally, a brief overview of psychiatric and medical interventions and a review of the etiology of rumination will be provided. The criteria for selecting articles for inclusion in this review was that the participant(s) was identified as having a developmental disability (e.g., autism, moderate mental retardation), b) the aberrant behavior targeted for reduction was either rumination or ruminative vomiting that occurred for no apparent organic reason, and c) one or more components of the intervention package were behavioral.

The literature search consisted of two components. Initially, computer searches of the psychological and medical literature using PsycINFO and Medline data-based systems were conducted. The descriptors rumination, vomiting, eating disorders, developmental disabilities, autism, and mental retardation were used. Secondly, the reference lists of the identified articles were reviewed to obtain articles not identified by the computer searches.

The forty studies identified have been placed initially into three categories based on the general characteristics of the intervention package (i.e., aversive, mildly aversive, and positive procedures). The published literature on the treatment acceptability of behavioral interventions for problem behaviors (e.g., stereotypy, self-injury) was used as a general guideline for the placement of the intervention package used in a study into one of the three possible categories (e.g., Witt, Elliott, and Martens, 1984). Within each of these three general intervention categories, the studies have been divided into groups based on common intervention components (e.g., extinction, overcorrection, differential reinforcement of other behavior). The groups are listed in alphabetical order within a category.

II. Etiology

Although the etiology of rumination is not completely understood by professionals in the fields of psychology, medicine, and developmental disabilities, several different theories have been discussed in the literature. In the early published literature (e.g., Peyer, 1685), most authors describe rumination as an atavistic analogy to the ruminative behaviors of herbivorous animals, particicularly cows (see, Gould, 1981 pp.124-145; Kanner, 1936; Parry-Jones, 1994).

In the psychiatric literature, a psycho-dynamic model has been most commonly used to describe the cause of rumination. According to this model, rumination results from a disruption of the mother-child relationship. That is, a child's mother rejects the child due to being either immature and/or because of her inability to fulfill an adult psycho-sexual role.

The rejected child then seeks internal gratification through their ruminative behavior. Psycho-dynamic intervention approaches typically have involved the use of intensive-mother procedures (e.g., increased holding, fondling, non-contingent attention) designed to repair the mother-child relationship. Several published studies have suggested that psycho-dynamic interventions might be effective (Berlin, McCullough, Liska, and Szurek, 1957; Richmond, Eddy, and Green, 1958); however, the lack of the use of well-controlled experimental designs makes it difficult to rule out the influence of extraneous variables and to reach confident conclusions about the efficacy of psycho-dynamic interventions.

According to a behavioral model, ruminative behavior can be explained in terms of basic behavioral principals (i.e., reinforcement [both positive and negative], stimulus control, and punishment). Applied behavior analysts, for example, have hypothesized that the rumination of persons with developmental disabilities is maintained by social-positive reinforcement in terms of attention from other people, social-negative reinforcement in the form of escape from instructional demands, or automatic reinforcement (e.g., the positive internal feedback produced by engaging in rumination).

III. Medical Information

A. Pathophysiology

The mechanism by which rumination occurs in humans is a subject of debate in the published literature. Retrograde peristalsis, present in animals that ruminate, is not present in humans (Malcom, 1997). Medical researchers have suggested the mechanism for rumination in humans is lower esophageal relaxation accompanied by increased intra-abdominal pressure, which allows food to pass through the esophagus into the mouth (O'Brien, Bruce, and Camilleri, 1995). Others researchers have suggested that rumination is an adaptation of the belch reflex (O'Brien, Bruce, and Camilleri, 1995).

B. Medical Diagnosis

Rumination can be difficult to diagnose, especially in persons with developmental disabilities, who often lack the communication skills necessary to describe and explain their own behavior. A retrospective review of the records of 147 children and adolescents with rumination, most without a developmental disability, showed that for those children obtaining an accurate diagnosis of rumination took an average of 2.1 years, during which time many of the individuals underwent extensive, costly, and invasive testing and interventions, with frequent misdiagnosis (Chial et al., 2003).

Some researchers have suggested that rumination can be diagnosed clinically based on history and absence of structural disease in adolescents and adults who are not developmentally disabled (O'Brien, Bruce and Camilleri, 1995). Thirty-eight adults and adolescents of average intellectual development participated in this retrospective record review. One common symptom of rumination identified included repetitive regurgitation of undigested or partly digested food that was not sour or bitter in taste, starting within minutes of a meal, and lasting 1-2 hours. Rumination also was described as being effortless and rarely associated with retching. Associated symptoms, reported with varying frequency, included weight loss, abdominal pain, constipation, diarrhea, bloating, and dental problems (Chial et al., 2003, Khan et al, 2000). Additionally, the results of Chial et al. (2003) found that during a 24 hour PH probe, individuals of average intellectual functioning with rumination had numerous brief episodes of reflux postprandially, but no significant episodes during sleep or supine positioning, as is typically seen in individuals with Gastroesophageal-Reflux Disease. Thereby, confirming O'Brien, Bruce and Camilleri's (1995) conclusion that rumination is a distinctively different disorder than gastroesophageal reflux disease in persons in the average range of intellectual functioning.

Table 1. Differential diagnosis/ medical conditions that may contribute to rumination in individuals with developmental disability:

Oral-motor disorders	Delayed swallow reflex Hyperactive gag reflex Oropharyngeal dysphagia
Esophageal/ Gastrointestinal Disorders	Aerophagia Congenital anatomic defects (pharyngeal diverticula) Delayed gastric emptying Esophageal stricture Esophagitis Gastroesophageal reflux disease Gastroparesis Hiatal Hernia Peptic ulcer disease, duodenal ulcer Pseudo-obstruction Pyloric Stenosis Small bowel obstruction Tracheoesophageal fistula
Infection	Heliobacter pylori infection
Medication side effects	Anticholinergics (dry mouth, muscle weakness) Anticonvulsants (dyspepsia) Benzodiazepines (drooling, dysphagia, decreased pharyngeal peristalsis) Digitalis (anxiety, mental disturbance) Chemotherapy (nausea, vomiting) Neuroleptics (Swallowing, esophageal function problems, pharyngeal dystonia)
Metabolic or Endocrine Disorders	Diabetes mellitus Inborn errors of metabolism Electrolyte Imbalance
Nervous System Disorders	CNS infection Hydrocephalus/ VP shunt malfunction
Psychiatric disorders	Depression Anxiety

The medical literature suggests that, in persons with developmental disabilities, other medical conditions may play a larger role in rumination behavior. Numerous studies have documented high rates of gastroesophageal reflux (GER) disease in individuals with intellectual disability and rumination symptoms. Bohmer et al. (1999), for example, found a rate of GER of almost 50%, in institutionalized individuals with an IQ less than 50. There was a strong correlation between vomiting, rumination, and diagnosis of GER. High incidence of Helicobacter pylori infection also has been found in adults with developmental disabilities, especially those in institutional settings (Wallace, Webb, and Schluter, 2002). Problem behavior and H. Pylori infection have been associated, although a treatment study failed to demonstrate behavioral or functional improvement following H. Pylori eradication (Wallace, Schluter, and Webb, 2004). This suggests that problem behavior may be a risk factor rather than a reversible consequence of H. pylori infection.

A study of 23 persons with severe developmental disabilities who lived in a large residential facility found that the majority of the participants had medical conditions, most notably gastroesophageal function problems that might contribute to their rumination (Rogers et al, 1992). The results of a videofluoroscopic swallow study and esophogram found significant gastroesophageal abnormalities that might contribute to rumination in 91% of the participants.

Gastroesophageal abnormalities identified included delayed initiation of the swallow reflex, Zenker diverticulum, esophageal dysmotility, aspiration, and hiatal hernia. Additionally, 43% of the persons who participated were receiving medications that might influence deglutition and gastroesophageal function, including benzodiazepines, neuroleptics, anticholinergics, and barbiturates. Rogers et al.'s (1992) results suggest that a more thorough medical evaluation of etiologies of ruminative behavior is required for individuals with developmental disabilities than those with typical cognitive functioning.

C. Medical and Surgical Treatment of Rumination

A review of the medical literature found little empirical support for the use of medications to reduce the rumination of typically developing individuals or individuals with developmental disabilities. A study of 147 persons, the majority of whom were in the average range of intellectual functioning, found that 53% of the participants had been prescribed medications for their rumination (included acid-blocking medications (N=66), prokinetic medications (N=56), acid-blocking plus prokinetic medications (N=47), anti-emetic medications (N=12), anti-depressants (N=10), and narcotic-pain medications (N=3) and that the medications had not produced a clinically significant improvement in any of the participants (Chial et al, 2003). Additionally, none of these medications have been described in the published literature as producing a clinically significant reduction in the rumination of persons with developmental disabilities. Medications that are used for the management of secondary vomiting such as phenothiazines (e.g., Thorazine and Haldol), antihistamines, steroids, cannaboids, and antiemetic drugs have been found to have little efficacy in reducing the rumination of persons with developmental disabilities (Starin and Fuqua, 1987). Although no clinically significant improvement in rumination with medication intervention has been reported in the published literature, one article, Kuruvilla and Trewby (1989) suggests that due to the difficult of diagnosing and treating rumination in persons with the developmental disabilities and the increased likelihood these individuals having related medical conditions, a trial of antacids and other anti-reflux medication should be considered whenever medical evaluations suggest that they are clinically appropriate. This recommendation, in our opinion, warrants further investigation by professionals who work with persons with developmental disabilities who display rumination.

Table 2. Behavioral Interventions to Reduce the Rumination of Persons with Developmental Disabilities

Reference	Participants	Setting	Intervention package	Functional Assessment or Analysis	Experimental Design	Generalization Data	Maintenance Data
Aversive Procedures							
Contingent Aversive Presentations							
Simpson & Sasso, 1978	10-year-old boy with mental retardation	Institution for persons with developmental disabilities	Contingent on rumination, the participant was verbally reprimanded and forced to swallow vomitus. 15-20 ml. of lemon juice also squirted in mouth. Participants lips and mouth area washed with soap and water for 30 sec. and facial cream massaged into lips and mouth area for 45 sec.	None reported	• BAB	None reported	None reported
Singh, 1979	4.8 year-old profoundly retarded boy	Institution for persons with developmental disabilities	Initially, 5 to 10 ml. of lemon juice was provided contingent on the occurrence of rumination. After the effects of lemon juice failed to maintain a reduction in rumination, 5 to 10 ml. of pepper sauce was provided contingent on rumination.	None reported	ABAC	None reported	12-month follow-up
	6-year-old profoundly retarded boy		Pepper sauce in the mouth provided contingent on the initial link of the response chain of rumination	None reported	ABAB	None reported	None reported

Table 2. Continued

Reference	Participants	Setting	Intervention package	Functional Assessment or Analysis	Experimental Design	Generalization Data	Maintenance Data
Aversive Procedures							
Contingent Aversive Presentations							
Marholin, Luiselli, Robinson, & Lott, 1980	16-year-old male with profound mental retardation	Institution for persons with developmental disabilities	5-10 cc. of lemon juice squirted in mouth contingent on rumination or placing fingers in mouth	None reported	Treatment only data	None reported	9 month follow-up
	11-year-old male with profound mental retardation	Institution for persons with developmental disabilities	5-10 cc. of lemon juice squirted in mouth and a contingent verbal reprimand provided contingent on rumination (treat # 1). 2-3 drops of Tabasco sauce in mouth contingent on rumination and social attention (e.g., "Good Job") contingent on the absence of rumination (treat # 2)		Treatment only data		70 day follow-up
Mestre, Resnick, & Berman, 1983	16-week-old male with developmental delays	Hospital	3 cc. of vinegar with 3 drops of Tabasco sauce contingent on rumination.	Authors suggest that behavior maintained by automatic reinforcement	Treatment only data	None reported	1 and 2 month follow-ups. 1 year follow-up.
Glasscock, Friman, O'Brien, & Christophersen, 1986	13-year-old female with Batten's disease and mental retardation	Institution for persons with developmental disabilities	2-5 ml. of lemon juice in mouth contingent on gagging	None reported	ABAB reversal design	Across meals	1, 3, and 7 month follow-ups

Table 2. Continued

Reference	Participants	Setting	Intervention package	Functional Assessment or Analysis	Experimental Design	Generalization Data	Maintenance Data
Aversive Procedures							
Contingent Electric Shock							
White & Tayor, 1967	23-year old female with severe mental retardation. 14-year-old male with profound mental retardation	Institution for persons with developmental disabilities	Contingent electric shock	None reported	Treatment only data	None reported	None reported
Luckey, Watson, & Musik, 1968	6-year-old male with severe mental retardation	Institution for persons with developmental disabilities	Contingent electric shock	None reported	Treatment only data	None reported	None reported
Bright & Whaley, 1968	11-year-old male with severe mental retardation	Institution for persons with developmental disabilities	Contingent electric shock	None reported	Treatment only data	None reported	None reported
Galbraith, Byrick, & Rutledge, 1970	13.5-year-old-male with severe mental retardation	Institution for persons with developmental disabilities	Contingent electric shock	None reported	Treatment only data	None reported	20 year follow-up reported by Svec et al. 1990.
Kohlenberg, 1970	7-year-old girl with severe mental retardation	Institution for persons with developmental disabilities	Contingent electric shock	None reported	AB design	None reported	None reported
Watkins, 1972	14-year-old boy with severe mental retardation	Institution for persons with developmental disabilities	Contingent electric shock	None reported	AB design	None reported	None reported
Wright & Thalassinos, 1973	4-year-old girl with severe mental retardation	Hospital	Contingent electric shock	None reported	AB design	None reported	6-month follow-up

Table 2. Continued

Reference	Participants	Setting	Intervention package	Functional Assessment or Analysis	Experimental Design	Generalization Data	Maintenance Data
Aversive Procedures							
Contingent Exercise							
Daniel, 1982	10 year-old male with profound mental retardation	Institution for persons with developmental disabilities	Brief contingent exercise and DRO	None reported	AB design	None reported	6 month follow-up
Overcorrection							
Azrin & Wesolwski, 1975	36-year-old female with profound mental retardation	Institution for persons with developmental disabilities	Required relaxation, time-out, and overcorrection all were evaluated. Neither relaxation nor time-out produced a clinically significant reduction in vomiting. Overcorrection reduced the behavior successfully.	None reported	ABCD	None reported	1, 4, and 52 week follow-ups
Duker & Seys, 1977	19-year-old female with profound mental retardation	Institution for persons with developmental disabilities	Positive-practice overcorrection and correction. Contingent on vomiting, the participant was required to wash her face with cold water and clean the area where she vomited (e.g., the floor). After she cleaned up, the participant was required to change her clothes	None reported	ABABAB	None reported	2-month follow-up

Table 2. Continued

Reference	Participants	Setting	Intervention package	Functional Assessment or Analysis	Experimental Design	Generalization Data	Maintenance Data
Aversive Procedures							
Contingent Exercise							
Foxx, Snyder, & Schroeder, 1979	25-year old male with profound mental retardation 22-year old female with profound mental retardation	Institution for persons with developmental disabilities	Oral-hygiene overcorrection and satiation	None reported	Multiple baseline across subjects design	Across meals	16-week follow-up
Singh, Manning, & Angell, 1982	Two 17-year-old male twins with profound mental retardation	Institution for persons with developmental disabilities	Contingent on rumination, participant was told "No" and required to brush his teeth for 2 min with Listerine and wipe his face with a washcloth.	None reported	Multiple baseline design across participants and meals	Fingers in mouth and tongue out behaviors increased slightly. Appropriate social behavior was found to decrease for part #1. Appropriate social behavior was found to increase for part #2	6-month follow-up

Table 2. Continued

Reference	Participants	Setting	Intervention package	Functional Assessment or Analysis	Experimental Design	Generalization Data	Maintenance Data
Mildly Aversive							
Extinction							
Wolf, Birnbrauer, Williams, & Lawler, 1965	9 year-old female with mental retardation	Institution for persons with developmental disabilities	The participant was not allowed to escape from her class and return to her dormitory contingent on the occurrence of vomiting	A functional assessment was conducted. Vomiting hypnotized to be maintained by social-negative reinforcement in the form of escape from demands	Treatment only design	Across settings	None reported
Smith & Lyon, 1976	25-year-old female with profound mental retardation	Institution for persons with developmental disabilities	Contingent on the absence of vomiting, social attention was provided. Contingent on vomiting, the participant was ignored for 30 min.	None reported	AB design	None reported	None reported
Time-out							
Smeets, 1970	18-year-old male with profound mental retardation	Institution for persons with developmental disabilities	Contingent removal of food. Window blinds and door of room closed contingent on rumination. Nurse left room for 30 min	None reported	Treatment only data	None reported	None reported
Response Cost							
Davis, Wieseler, & Hanzel, 1983	26-year-old male with profound mental retardation	Institution for persons with developmental disabilities	Contingent on the occurrence of rumination bluegrass music was terminated and participant was verbally reprimanded.	None reported	Multiple-baseline across times of day	Intervention generalized across settings and behavior change agents	None reported

Table 2. Continued

Reference	Participants	Setting	Intervention package	Functional Assessment or Analysis	Experimental Design	Generalization Data	Maintenance Data
Positive Procedures							
Differential Reinforcement							
Mullick, Schroeder, & Rojahn, 1980 *	15-year-old male with profound mental retardation	Inpatient treatment unit (i.e. self-injurious behavior program at Murdoch Center)	Experimental analysis in which DRO, DRI, Extinction and DRI, and Extinction were compared. DRI found to be more effective than DRO	None reported	Latin Square design	Data on various collateral behaviors were examined (e.g., tongue out, hand in mouth). None were found to be significantly correlated with vomiting	Not applicable
Conrin, Pennypacker, Johnston, & Rast, 1982	23-year-old male with profound mental retardation 19-year-old male with profound mental retardation	Institution for persons with developmental disabilities	Small pieces of Cookie or bits of peanut butter were provided contingent on the absence of rumination	None reported	ABCDAC (part # 1) ABCDEFADEF (part #2)	None reported	
McKeegan, Estill, & Campbell, 1987	23-year-old male with severe mental retardation and autism	Day-treatment program	Controlled eating program that consisted of having the participant eat smaller bites of food. Thus, extending the amount of time it took to eat a meal. Contingent on not engaging in rumination within 2 min interval and being on-task at the end of the interval, the participant received a small low calorie edible (e.g., piece of popcorn) and verbal praise	None reported	A-B-A-B-BC-B-BC withdrawal design	None reported	6-month follow-up

Table 2. Continued

Reference	Participants	Setting	Intervention package	Functional Assessment or Analysis	Experimental Design	Generalization Data	Maintenance Data
Positive Procedures							
Satiation							
Jackson, Johnson, Ackron, & Crowley, 1975	29-year-old male with profound mental retardation 27-year-old male with profound mental retardation	Institution for persons with developmental disabilities	Both participants were allowed to eat all the food that they could consume. The first participant was provided double portions of each meal plus extra cereal, ice cream, and milk shakes. The second participant was provided with extra portions of his soft diet.	None reported	ABAB (part #1) ABA (part #2)	None reported	10 day follow-up
Libby & Phillips, 1978	Male with profound mental retardation	Institution for persons with developmental disabilities	Extra portions of food provided	None reported	AB design	None reported	3 month follow-up
Borreson & Anderson, 1982	21-year-old male with profound mental retardation	Institution for persons with developmental disabilities	A comparison between satiation, satiation with time out from music, and satiation with time out from music and tactile stimulation was conducted. Satiation with time out from music and tactile stimulation was found to be the most effective procedure.	None reported	ABCDADAED design	None reported	None reported

Table 2. Continued

Reference	Participants	Setting	Intervention package	Functional Assessment or Analysis	Experimental Design	Generalization Data	Maintenance Data
Positive Procedures							
Satiation							
Rast, Johnston, Drum, Conrin, 1981*	19-year-old male with severe mental retardation 21-year-old male with profound mental retardation 24-year-old male with profound mental retardation	Institution for persons with developmental disabilities	The relationship between the quantity of food ingested and rumination was examined. Rumination was demonstrated to decrease when large quantities of food were ingested.	Not applicable	Experimental analysis using a parametric design	Not applicable	Not applicable
Rast, Johnston, & Drum, 1984*	22-year-old female with profound mental retardation 34-year-old male with profound mental retardation 32-year-old male with profound mental retardation	Institution for persons with developmental disabilities	The control of rumination by the quantity of food eaten at meals was examined. Rumination was demonstrated to decrease when food quantity increased and increased when food quantity decreased.	Not applicable	Experimental analysis using a parametric design	Not applicable	Not applicable

Table 2. Continued

Reference	Participants	Setting	Intervention package	Functional Assessment or Analysis	Experimental Design	Generalization Data	Maintenance Data
Positive Procedures							
Satiation							
Rast, Johnston, Allen, & Drum, 1985*	34 year-old male with profound mental retardation 23-year-old female with profound mental retardation 22-year-old female with profound mental retardation 18 year-old female with profound mental retardation	Institution for persons with developmental disabilities	Examined the properties of food that influence the relationship between quantity of food ingested and rumination. A starch-satiation procedure was only found to be effective when the participants were permitted to consume unlimited quantities of food.	Not applicable	Experimental analysis using a parametric design	Not applicable	Not applicable
Rast, Ellinger-Allen, & Johnston, 1985*	Four males with profound mental retardation	Institution for persons with developmental disabilities	The relationship between meal size and rumination was examined. Reduction of rumination was associated with large dietary increases and being allowed to eat until a satiation criteria was reached.	Not applicable	Experimental analysis using a parametric design	Not applicable	Not applicable

Table 2. Continued

Reference	Participants	Setting	Intervention package	Functional Assessment or Analysis	Experimental Design	Generalization Data	Maintenance Data
Positive Procedures							
Satiation							
Lobato, Carlson, & Barrera, 1986*	28-year-old female with profound mental retardation 25-year-old male with severe mental retardation	Institution for persons with developmental disabilities	After participants had eaten the regular portions of their standard meals, they were offered unlimited quantities of two or more low calorie foods (e.g., fruit, vegetables). Participants also offered unlimited quanaties of low calorie foods between meals	Rumination was described as being maintained by automatic reinforcement	Multiple baseline across subjects with embedded withdrawal design	Effects of satiation on stereotypic behavior was examined. No generalization across behaviors was demonstrated	None reported
Johnston, Greene, Vazin, Wiston, & Rawal, 1990*	Three persons with profound mental retardation who ranged in age from 25 to 36 years	Institution for persons with developmental disabilities	A comparison between puree meals and meals of a normal consistency was conducted. An increase in rumination was associated with puree meals	Not applicable	ABAB design	Not applicable	Not applicable

Table 2. Continued

Reference	Participants	Setting	Intervention package	Functional Assessment or Analysis	Experimental Design	Generalization Data	Maintenance Data
Positive Procedures							
Satiation							
Greene, Johnston, Rossi, Rawal, Winston, & Barron, 1991*	53-year-old male with profound mental retardation 31-year-old female with profound mental retardation 37-year-old male with profound mental retardation 45-year-old male with profound mental retardation 22-year-old male with severe mental retardation	Institution for persons with developmental disabilities	The effect of peanut butter on the rates of rumination was examined. Both the caloric density and consistency of the peanut butter was manipulated. An inverse relationship between the rate of rumination and amount of peanut butter eaten was found. This result was found to be determined mainly by an increase in calories. A smaller effect was associated with the consistency of peanut butter	Not applicable	Various within subject single subject comparisons (e.g., AB, ABA, ABCDEA)	Not applicable	Not applicable
Clauser & Scibak, 1990	22-year-old male with profound mental retardation 33-year-old male with profound mental retardation 40 year old male with profound mental retardation	Institution for persons with developmental disabilities	Triple portions of food of regular consistency and unlimited bowls of cold cereal with milk provided during each scheduled meal. Satiation was defined as 2 consecutive min. of declining to eat in the presence of food.	None reported	ABA Design (part # 1) ABAB design (part # 2) ABAB design (part # 3)	A collateral reduction in self-injury (part # 1 and 2) or stereotypy (part # 3) was observed	6 month and 2 year follow-ups (part # 3).

Table 2. Continued

Reference	Participants	Setting	Intervention package	Functional Assessment or Analysis	Experimental Design	Generalization Data	Maintenance Data
Positive Procedures							
Satiation							
Luiselli, Medeiros, Jasinowski, Smith, & Cameron, 1994	15-year-old boy with autism	Residential school for persons with disabilities	Modified diet which included no tomato sauce, mixed vegetables, or apples. These food were observed to be associated with rumination and vomiting. Limited portions of meat. Extra snacks and portions of food during meals. To decrease mealtime anxiety, all meals were eaten in an area free of other students and their staff members. Contingent on rumination, the participant's staff members ignored the behavior. Contingent on vomiting, the participant was required to help clean-up the environment.	Rumination was hypnotized to be controlled by both internal (e.g., anxiety, automatic reinforcement) and external variables (e.g., social attention)	AB Design	Across settings and staff	1, 2, 3, and 4 month follow-ups

Table 2. Continued

Reference	Participants	Setting	Intervention package	Functional Assessment or Analysis	Experimental Design	Generalization Data	Maintenance Data
Positive Procedures							
Satiation							
Dunn, Lockwood, Williams, & Peacock, 1997	24-year-old man with profound mental retardation and Down syndrome	Institution for persons with developmenta l disabilities	Participant provided with unlimited access to high starch foods or fruits and vegetables, in addition to his regular meals	Functional assessment. Rumination was hypothized to be maintained by automatic reinforcement because the behavior was observed to occur independently of social-mediated consequences	ABAB withdrawal design with long-term follow-up	Across meals and staff	7-year follow-up
Wilder, Draper, Williams, & Higbee, 1997	46-year-old male with profound mental retardation and blindness	Group home located on residential campus	Initially, a comparison among a shower placement (an alternative high probability alternative behavior), satiation, and liquid rescheduling was conducted. The satiation procedure consisted of providing a teaspoonful of gelatin or pudding every 20 s during the 30 min after each meal. An analysis of whether or not rumination continued 60 min after the intervention was terminated was conducted.	Functional assessment. Rumination was hypnotized to be maintained by automatic reinforcement because the behavior was observed to occur independently of social-mediated consequences	ABAB withdrawal design with an embedded alternating-treatments design	None reported	None reported

Table 2. Continued

Reference	Participants	Setting	Intervention package	Functional Assessment or Analysis	Experimental Design	Generalization Data	Maintenance Data
Positive Procedures							
Satiation							
Thibadeau, Blew, Reeedy, & Luiselli, 1999	18-year old male with mental retardation and autistic features	Community-based group home for persons with developmental disabilities	White bread was provided noncontingently for 1 hour following each meal whenever the participant signed "eat"	None reported	ABCB withdrawal design	None reported	9, 12, and 15 month follow-ups
Dudley, Johnson, & Barnes, 2002	9-year-old girl with autism	Residential student in a community-based school for persons with disabilities	After the completion of each meal, the participant was provided access to two types of starchy food (e.g., cereal, pasta, rice cakes)	None reported	ABAB withdrawal design	Across meals	4 year follow-up

*=Studies in which an experimental analysis was conducted. These studies were included in the current review because the information obtain was judged to be important to professional conducting clinical research.

Surgical interventions also are frequently suggested for individuals with rumination. For individuals with clearly identifiable organic pathology such as gastroesophageal reflux, hiatal hernia, or bowel obstruction, surgical intervention is often successful in reducing ruminative behavior. In the absence of such diagnoses, however, surgical interventions such as antireflux surgeries or creating artificial closing mechanisms at the gastroesophageal junction generally result in limited, short-term improvement and high risk for long term surgical complications (Starin and Fuqua, 1987).

IV. Review of the Published Behavioral Literature

A. Participant Characteristics

Of the sixty-six people who participated in the studies reviewed, forty-seven were male and sixteen were female. The sex of three of the participants was not specified. Most of the participants had severe or profound mental retardation (N=59). The average age of the participants was 21.4 years with a range of 4 to 53 years of age. Table 2 provides more information on each participant's age, gender, and intellectual functioning.

B. Interventions

The interventions reviewed were categorized broadly into three groups. Within each group the interventions were further categorized based on common treatment characteristics. The most commonly used interventions where, in order, of frequency satiation (N=16), electric shock (N=7), aversive presentations (N=5), overcorrection (N=4), differential reinforcement (N=3), Extinction (N=2), contingent exercise (N=1), response cost (N=1), and time-out (N=1). A brief description of the intervention packages used in each of the studies reviewed is provided in the column labeled Intervention Package in Table 2.

C. Settings

Of the 40 experiments reviewed, 32 were conducted in institutional or residential settings for persons with developmental disabilities. Two of the studies were conducted in community-based residential settings. The remaining studies were conducted in segrated school settings, hospitals, or specialized treatment programs for aberrant behaviors.

D. Behavioral Function of Rumination

None of the authors of the studies reviewed conducted a functional analysis in order to identify the behavioral variables maintaining a participant's rumination. A functional analysis is an assessment protocol in which a person is systematically exposed to various situations in order to identify the variable(s) maintaining their problem behavior. The authors of several studies did describe the variables they believed were maintaining a participant's rumination based on their behavioral observations. Variables hypothesized to maintain a participant's rumination were, in order of frequency, automatic reinforcement N= 5, social-positive reinforcement (i.e. attention from other people) N= 1, and social-negative reinforcement (i.e., escape from instructional demands) N=1. None of the authors of the studies reviewed hypothesized that social positive reinforcement in the form of access to tangible items was maintaining a participant's rumination.

C. Generalization

None of the authors of the studies reviewed reported the use of systematic strategies (e.g., train loosely, sequential modification) to promote the generalization of the results obtained across settings, behavior change agents/people, or situations (e.g., a reduction in rumination from meal to snack time). In several studies, the degree to which an intervention package generalizes across situations (e.g., meals or behavior change agents) was evaluated, and these studies generally reported that the intervention package could be successfully implemented in additional settings with results similar to those obtained in the initial setting in which the intervention package was implemented.

V. Discussion

The above review of the published literature on behavioral intervention packages designed to reduce the rumination of persons with developmental disabilities has demonstrated that a variety of behavior intervention strategies have been used to reduce rumination successfully (e.g., contingent aversive presentations, differential reinforcement of other behavior). Additionally, the majority of the studies were conducted in institutional versus community-based settings. Finally, in the majority of the studies the researchers implemented the intervention versus other behavior change agents such as parents. The results of the literature review highlight several issues that require further discussion. Each of these issues is discussed below.

Researchers should include analogue -functional analyses in their research studies in order to identify the specific variables maintaining rumination.

In the future, researchers examining the efficacy of behavioral intervention packages to reduce rumination should include an analogue-functional analysis in order to identify the specific variables maintaining a participant's rumination. The published research reviewed for this chapter provides ambiguous information about the variables that maintain rumination. Observational data described by several of the authors suggest that environmental variables such as social attention are the most likely cause of rumination. However, data from studies in which non-contingently provided food has been used to reduce rumination suggest that automatic reinforcement (i.e., the internal feedback produced from engaging in the behavior) maybe the most likely variable maintaining rumination.

The analogue functional analysis protocol developed by Iwata and his colleagues in which a person is systematically exposed to various situations in order to determine whether or not a problem behavior is maintained by either environmental consequences (i.e., social attention from other people, escape from instructional demands, access to high-preference item or activities) or automatic reinforcement (i.e., the internal consequences produced by engaging in the behavior) might provide much useful information concerning the variables maintaining rumination. Identifying the specific cause of rumination may be critical to the successful development of intervention strategies for rumination because researchers have demonstrated that prescriptive function-based interventions are more likely to be reduce a problem behavior successfully than non-function based interventions. Additionally, data from analogue-functional analyses might contribute greatly to our understanding of the etiology of rumination, particularly the degree to which a behavioral-analytic model explains rumination.

A study conducted by Pizza, Hanley, and Fisher (1996) in which a functional analysis of pica, another eating disorder commonly displayed by persons with developmental disabilities, illustrates the potential contribution that the use of the analogue-functional analysis protocol might make to our understanding of rumination. Initially, it was demonstrated that the pica of a 17-year-old man with severe mental retardation was maintained by the availability of nicotine in cigarettes. During this assessment, several different conditions were examined within the framework of a single-subject alternating-treatments design. Each session was 10 min. in length and all sessions were conducted in a small room containing a one-way mirror. When a condition in which cigarette butts containing tobacco were available was compared to a condition in which herbal cigarette butts were available, the participant consumed more cigarette butts in the condition in which the butts containing tobacco were available suggesting that nicotine was the maintaining variable. A second functional analysis was conducted in which the consequences for the display of pica were systematically manipulated. During the social-attention condition, the participant was provided a magazine and he was verbally prompted to look at it. Contingent on the occurrence of pica, the participant was briefly verbally reprimanded. During the alone condition, which was designed to assess whether pica was internally maintained, the participant was left alone in a room containing six cigarette butts all containing tobacco and was observed through a one-way mirror. During the control condition, the participant was given several high-preference items (e.g., a ball) and social attention was provided by a therapist contingent on the absence of pica. The combined results of the functional analyses described above demonstrated that the participant's pica was internally maintained, specifically by nicotine. Based on the results of the functional analysis, the authors provided the participant with non-contingently provided food (a functional alternative behavior to the participant's pica) in the presence of a purple card. The purple card was demonstrated to have stimulus control over the participant's pica. That is, when the participant was given the purple card and told not to engage in pica, he did not display the behavior across a variety of natural settings, despite the availability of cigarette butts.

Researchers and practioners should follow the less-restrictive alternative approach when designing interventions to reduce rumination.

The majority of behavioral intervention packages that have been successfully demonstrated to reduce the rumination of persons with developmental disabilities have included a punishment-based intervention component. Of the forty-two studies reviewed, nineteen contained at least one punishment-based component. However, a recent trend in the published literature towards the publication of intervention packages based on positive procedures was shown by the results of the literature review conducted for this chapter. This trend in the published literature suggests that the principle of the least restrictive alternative has had an impact on the treatment selected. That is, the authors of the studies reviewed have attempted to treat the rumination of persons with developmental disabilities using positive procedures prior to the implementation of punishment-based strategies. This finding is important because the authors of several published studies have demonstrated that people view punishment-based behavioral intervention packages as being less socially valid than antecedent or positive reinforcement based intervention packages. Research that examines whether or not this trend in the published literature also is reflected in the clinical practice of various professionals who design and implement intervention packages in residential settings in which persons with developmental disabilities typically live is needed (e.g., community-based group homes).

Further replication of intervention packages used with persons who display rumination and are within the normal range of intellectual functioning are needed to determine whether or not these strategies are also effective with people with disabilities.

Researchers who work with person of average or above intellectual functioning who display rumination have demonstrated the efficacy of various intervention packages to reduce rumination. Professional who work with persons with developmental disabilities need to examine the degree to which these strategies also can be successfully used with persons with developmental disabilities. Weakley, Petti, and Karwisch (1997), for example, demonstrated that postmeal chewing of gum reduced the rumination of 15-year-old girl of average intellectual functioning who was hospitalized for the treatment of anorexia nervosa. Additionally, Donnelly and Olczak (1990) showed that the differential reinforcement of gum chewing with small amounts of coffee successfully reduced the pica of two men with profound mental retardation. The combined results of these studies suggest that the efficacy of postmeal chewing of gum on the rumination of person with developmental disabilities should be examined.

In a second example, Wagaman, Williams, and Michael (1998) demonstrated that a simplified habit-reversal intervention successfully reduced the rumination of a 6-year-old girl.. The habit-reversal intervention package consisted of three components: a) awareness training, b) the use of an incompatible behavior (i.e., diaphragmatic breathing), and c) social support provided by the girl's parents. Awareness training consisted of teaching the participant to self-monitor the occurrence of her rumination. Diaphragmtic breathing involved teaching the participant to make her abdomen rise and fall during breathing and making each breath last for a minimum of 3 seconds. Social support consisted of the girl's mother reminding her to use the self-monitoring and breathing procedures while providing her with positive reinforcement for compliance (e.g., social praise). Since researchers have demonstrated that habit-reversal can reduce the rumination of persons of normal intellectual functioning, researchers should examine whether or not it is an appropriate intervention for people with developmental disabilities who display rumination.

Additional Studies conducted in community-based settings in which many persons with developmental disabilities live are needed.

The majority of the studies that examine the efficacy of intervention packages to reduce rumination have been conducted in institutional settings. However, persons with developmental disabilities, including many people with severe and profound developmental disabilities, are living in community-based settings (e.g., a community-based group home, their parents' home) in increasing numbers. Therefore, more research studies need to be conducted in community-based settings in order to examine the external validity of the intervention package reviewed, particularly those intervention packages based on positive reinforcement (e.g. differential reinforcement) or antecedent manipulations (e.g., satiation).

Additional parent and staff training studies designed to teach parents and other professionals how to successfully implement behavioral intervention packages to reduce rumination are needed.

In the majority of the studies reviewed, the intervention was implemented by one of the experimenters. More research studies are needed that explore the efficacy of interventions to teach the parents of children with disabilities, staff members of community-based residential settings, and other professionals who work with persons with disabilities to implement behavior intervention strategies design to reduce rumination. Recently, published studies in the area of feeding problems provide an excellent model which needs to be replicated by professionals who work with persons with developmental disabilities who display rumination. McCartney, Anderson, and English (2005), for example, showed that parents of persons with disabilities can be taught to use escape extinction and differential reinforcement using video-modeling and direct observations with contingent verbal feedback to treat their children's feeding problems. The degree to which such training packages can be used to teach parents, teaching staff, and professionals who work with person with developmental disabilities who display rumination in community-based settings is needed.

The overall result of this review and analysis suggests several specific recommendations for both researchers and practitioners who work with development disabilities who display rumination. The successful implementation of these recommendations will, hopefully, further our understanding of rumination and result in the development of more potentially effective interventions to reduce the rumination of persons with developmental disabilities across a variety of settings.

References

Azrin, N. H., and Wesolowski, M. D. (1975). Eliminating habitual vomiting in a retarded adult by positive practice and self-correction. *Journal of Behavior Therapy and Experimental Psychiatry*, *6*, 145-148.

Bohmer, C. M., Niezen-de Boer, M. C., Klinkenberg-Knol, E. C., Deville, W.- M., Nadorp, J. H. S. M. and Meuwissen, S. M. (1999). The prevalence of gastroesophageal reflux disease in institutionalized intellectually disabled individuals. *The American Journal of Gastroenterology, 94,* 804-810.

Borreson, P. M., and Anderson, J. L. (1982). The elimination of chronic rumination through a combination of procedures. *Mental Retardation*, *20*, 34-38.

Barton, L. E., and Baron, C. L. (1985). An effective and benign treatment of rumination. *Journal of the Association for the Severely Handicapped*, 10, 168-171.

Bright, G. O., and Whaley, D. L. (1968). Suppression of regurgitation and rumination with aversive events. *Michigan Mental Health Research Bulletin, 2*, 17-20.

Clauser, B. and Scibak, J. W. (1990). Direct and generalized effects of food satiation in reducing rumination. *Research in Developmental Disabilities*. *11*, 23-36.

Conrin, J. Penneypacker, H.S., Johnston, J. and Rast, J. (1982). Differential reinforcement of other behavior to treat chronic rumination of mental retardates. *Journal of Behavioral Therapy and Experimental Psychiatry, 13*, 325-329.

Daniel, W. (1982). Management of chronic rumination with a contingent exercise procedure employing topographically dissimilar behavior. *Journal of Behavioral Therapy and Experimental Psychiatry, 13*, 149-152.

Davis, W. B., Wieseler, N. A., and Hanzel, T. E. (1983). Reduction of rumination and out-of-seat behavior and generalization of treatment effects using a non-intrusive method. *Journal of Music Therapy, 20*, 115-131.

Duker, P. C. and Seys, D. M. (1977). Elimination of vomiting in a retarded female using restitutional overcorrection. *Behavior Therapy, 8*, 255-257.

Dunn, J., Lockwood, K., Williams, D.E., and Peacock, S. (1997). A seven year follow-up of treating rumination with dietary satiation. *Behavioral Interventions, 12*, 163-172.

Dudley, L. L., Johnson, C., and Barnes, R. S. (2002). Decreasing rumination using a starchy food satiation procedure.

Foxx, R.M., Snyder, M. S., and Schroeder, F. (1979). A food satiation and oral hygiene punishment program to suppress chronic rumination by retarded persons. *Journal of Autism and Developmental Disorders, 9*, 399-412.

Galbraith, D. A., Byrick, R. J., and Rutledge, J. T. (1970). An aversive conditioning approach to the inhibition of chronic vomiting. *Canadian Psychiatric Association Journal, 15*, 311-313.

Glasscock, S. G., Friman, P. C., O'Brien, S., and Christophersen, E. R. (1986). Varied citrus treatment of ruminant gagging in a teenager with Batten's disease. *Journal of Behavior Therapy and Experimental Psychiatry, 17*, 129-133.

Greene, K. S., Johnston, J. M., Rossi, M., Rawal, A., Winston, M., and Barron, S. (1991). Effects of peanut butter on ruminating. *American Journal of Mental Retardation, 95*, 631-645.

Heering, P. W., Wilder, D. A., and Ladd, C. (2003). Liquid rescheduling for the treatment of rumination. *Behavioral Interventions, 18*, 199-207.

Jackson, G. M., Johnson, C. R., Ackron, G. S., and Crowley, R. (1975). Food satiation as a procedure to decelerate vomiting. *American Journal of Mental Deficiency, 80*, 223-227.

Johnson, J. M., Greene, K. S., Rawal, A., Varzin, T. and Winston, M. (1991). Effects of caloric level on ruminating. *Journal of Applied Behavior Analysis, 24*, 597-603.

Johnson, J. M., Greene, K. S., Varzin, T., Winston, M., Rawal, A., and Chuang, S. (1990). Effects of food consistency on rumination. *The Psychological Record, 40*, 609-618.

Johnson, J.M., and Greene, K. S., (1992). Relation between rumination and quantity of food consumed. *Mental Retardation, 30*, 7-11.

Kohlenber, R. J. (1970). The punishment of persistent vomiting: a case study. *Journal of Applied Behavior Analysis, 3*, 241-245.

Libby, D. G. and Phillips, E. (1978). Eliminating rumination behavior in a profoundly retarded adolescent. An exploratory study. *Mental Retardation.* 16, 57.

Lobato, E., Carlson, E. I., and Barrera, R. D. (1986). Modified satiation reducing ruminative vomiting without excessive weight gain. *Applied Research in Mental Retardation*, 7, 337-347.

Luckey, R. E., Watson, C. M., and Musick, J. K., (1968). Aversive conditioning as a means of inhibiting vomiting and rumination. *American Journal of Mental Deficiency, 73*, 139-142.

Luiselli, J. K., Medeiros, J., Jasinowski, C., Smith, A., and Cameron, M. J. (1994). Behavioral medicine treatment of ruminative vomiting and associated weight loss in an adolescent with autism. *Journal of Autism and Developmental Disorders, 24*, 619-629.

Marholin, D., Luiselli, J. K., Robinson, M., and Lott, I. T. (1980). Response contingent taste aversion in treating chronic ruminative vomiting of institutionalized profoundly retarded children. *Journal of Mental Deficiency Research*, 24, 47-55.

Masalsky, C. J., and Luiselli, J. K. (1998). Brief report: effects of supplemental feedings on white bread on chronic rumination. *Behavioral Interventions, 13*, 227-223.

Mestre, J. R., Resnick, R. J., Wallace, F., and Berman, M.D. (1983). Behavior modification in the treatment of rumination. *Clinical Pediatrics, 22*, 488-491.

McKeegan, G. F., Estill, K., and Campbell, B. (1987). Elimination of rumination by controlled eating and differential reinforcement. *Journal of Behavioral Therapy and Experimental Psychiatry, 18*, 143-148.

Mulick, J. A. Schroeder, S. R. and Rojahn, J. (1980). Chronic ruminative vomiting: a comparison of four treatment procedures. *Journal of Autism and Developmental Disorders, 10*, 203-213.

O'Neil, P. M., White, J. L., King, C. R., and Carek, D. J. (1979). Controlling childhood rumination through differential reinforcement of other behavior. *Behavior Modification, 3*, 355-372.

Rast, J. Ellinger-Allen, J. A., and Johnston, J. M. (1985). Dietary management of rumination: four case studies. *The American Journal of Clinical Nu*trition, *42*, 95-101.

Rast, J. Johnston, J. M., and Drum, C. (1984). A parametric analysis of the relationship between food quantity and rumination. *Journal of the Experimental Analysis of Behavior, 41*, 125-134.

Rast, J. Johnston, J. M., Ellinger-Allen, J., and Drum, C. (1985). Effects of nutritional and mechanical properties of food on ruminative behavior. *Journal of the Experimental Analysis of Behavior, 44*, 195-206.

Rast, J., Johnson, J. M., Drum, C. and Conrin, J. (1981). The relation of food quantity to rumination behavior. *Journal of Applied Behavior Analysis*, 14, 121-130.

Simpson, R. L., and Sasso. G. M. (1978). The modification of rumination in a severely emotionally disturbed child through an overcorrection procedure. *AAESPH Review*, 145-150.

Singh, N. N. (1979). Aversive control of rumination in the mentally retarded. *Journal of Practical Approaches to Developmental Handicap, 3*, 2-6.

Singh, N. N., Manning, P. J., and Angell, M. J. (1982). Effects of an oral hygiene punishment procedure on chronic rumination and collateral behaviors in monozygous twins. *Journal of Applied Behavior Analysis, 15*, 309-314.

Smeets, P. M. (1970). Withdrawal of social reinforcers as a means of controlling rumination and regurgitation in a profoundly retarded person. Training School Bulletin, 67, 158-163.

Smith, D. W., and Lyon, R. (1976). Eliminating vomiting behavior in a profoundly retarded resident. *Research and the Retarded*, 3, 24-27.

Thibadeau, S., Blew, P., Reedy, P., and Luiselli, J. K. (1999). Access to white bread as an intervention for chronic ruminative vomiting. *Journal of Behavior therapy and Experimental Psychiatry*, *30*, 137-144.

Wagaman, J. R., Williams, D. E., and Camilleri, M. (1998). Behavioral intervention of the treatment of rumination. *Journal of Pediatric Gastroenterology and Nutrition*. *27*, 596-598.

Wallace, R. A., Webb, P. M. and Schluter, P. J. (2002). Environmental, medical, behavioral and disability factors associated with Helicobacter pylori infection in adults with intellectual disability. *Journal of Intellectual Disability Research*, *46*, 51-60.

Wallace, R. A., Webb, P. M. and Schluter, P. J. (2004). Effects of Helicobacter pylori eradication among adults with intellectual disability. *Journal of Intellectual Disability Research*, *48*, 646-654.

Watkins, J. T. (1972). Treatment of chronic vomiting and extreme emaciation by an aversive stimulus: a case study. *Psychological Reports*, *31*, 803-805.

Weakley, M., Petti, T., and Karwish, G. (1997). Case study: chewing gum treatment of rumination in an adolescent with an eating disorder. *Journal of the American Academy of Child and Adolescent Psychiatry*, 36, 1124-1127.

White, J. C., and Taylor, D. J. (1967). Noxious conditioning as a treatment for rumination. *Mental Retardation*, *5*, 30-33.

Wilder, D. A., Draper, R., Williams, W. L, and Higbee, T. S. (1997). A comparison of noncontingent reinforcement, other competing stimulation, and liquid rescheduling for the treatment of rumination. *Behavioral Interventions*, *12*, 55-64.

Winton, A. S. and Singh, N. N. (1983). Rumination in pediatric populations: a behavioral analysis. *Journal of the American Academy of Child Psychiatry*, *22*, 269-275.

Witt, J. C., Elliott, S. N., and Martens, B. K. (1984). Accetpability of behavioral interventions used in classrooms: The influence of amount of teacher time, severity of behavior problem, and type of intervention. *Behavioral Disorders*, *9*, 95-104.

Wolf, M. M., Birnbrauer, J., Lawler, J., and William, T. (1970). The operant extinction, reinstatement and re-extinction of vomiting behavior in a retarded child. In R. Ulrich, T., Statnik, and J. Mabry (Eds.), *Control of human behavior: From cure to prevention* (vol 2, pp 364-366). Glenview, Ill: Scott Foresman.

Wright, L., and Thalassinos, P. A. (1973). Success with electric shock in habitual vomiting: Report of two cases in young children. *Clinical Pediatrics*, *12*, 594-597.

In: Eating Disorders and Weight Loss Research
Editor: Jerome S. Rubin, pp. 105-125
ISBN 1-60021-334-0

Chapter 5

A New Carbohydrate Marker of Eating Behaviors in Eating Disorders

Daisuke Yasuhara, Tetsuro Naruo and Akio Inui
Department of Behavioral Medicine, Kagoshima University
Graduate School of Medical and Dental Sciences,
8-35-1 Sakuragaoka, Kagoshima-City, 890-8520, Japan

Abstract

Patients with eating disorders (EDs) are secretive with regard to their eating behaviors, and clinicians often experience difficulty in assessing their status using interviews or self-reported questionnaires. Although evaluations of clinical status should be made during treatment, few biological markers of eating behaviors in patients with anorexia nervosa and bulimia nervosa have been identified. Thus, the development of more useful markers is required in order to ensure successful treatment. In previous research on EDs, carbohydrate metabolism appeared to be associated with nutritional status; however, carbohydrate markers with which to assess eating behaviors remained to be identified. This chapter explores the relationship between carbohydrate metabolism and eating behaviors in these patients, and presents recent research on a new carbohydrate marker, the insulinogenic index at 15 minutes, which precisely mirrors eating behaviors in patients with EDs. The authors also address the clinical significance of assessing eating behaviors in patients with EDs from the biological perspective and discuss future directions in the field.

Introduction

Eating disorders (EDs), especially anorexia nervosa (AN) and bulimia nervosa (BN), are psychiatric disorders characterized by abnormal eating behaviors (e.g., severe energy restriction, binge eating, and vomiting) and various mental and physical complications [1]. The increasing prevalence in young female populations (AN 0.7%; BN, 1% to 2%) and long-term poor prognosis are serious problems associated with these disorders [2, 3]. However, there are considerable difficulties in assessing patients' conditions or correcting their abnormal eating behaviors, because the core psychopathology of these disorders is associated with an intense fear of obesity and patients often manipulate their self-reported conditions.

With regard to anorexia nervosa, recent studies of long-term prognosis have revealed that this disorder diminishes quality of life among adolescents and young adults [4, 5]. Although weight gain during hospitalization is an important prognostic factor for disease outcome [5], patients with AN are ambivalent about treatment and often exhibit treatment resistance or refusal. Since the characteristic psychopathology in AN may closely relate to severe starvation, some therapists emphasize the need for a careful nutritional assessment and the formulation of a nutritional program before other strategies are attempted [6, 7]. However, it is very difficult for clinicians to accurately assess the progress of the nutritional status of patients using interviews or self-reported body weight measurement during treatment, because patients often manipulate body weight measurements, especially during periods of distinct fear of obesity [8]. These problems could be associated with the poor treatment progress often seen in these patients. Thus, it is clinically important that investigations seek to identify a useful biological marker for assessing patients' conditions, particularly the progress of refeeding during nutritional rehabilitation.

In terms of bulimia nervosa, patients follow a chaotic eating behavior pattern, with periods of severe energy restriction, binge eating, and compensatory vomiting [9]. For these patients, evaluations of the stability of eating behavior should be made in the course of treatment. However, in most cases, patients with BN are secretive with regard to their eating behavior, and clinicians face difficulties in accurately assessing a patient's status using interviews or self-reported questionnaires [9]. Although several markers of nutritional status or vomiting activity have been reported [10-22], few useful biological markers can be used to assess the stability of eating behavior in BN. Therefore, investigations to define a useful marker for assessing the stability of eating behavior (body weight maintenance and vomiting activity) are also clinically important.

Previous studies on EDs have shown various abnormalities in carbohydrate metabolism prior to therapeutic interventions, most of which were reversible after weight restoration or treatment. Thus, this chapter explores the relationship between carbohydrate metabolism and eating behaviors (weight restoration in AN, and body weight maintenance and vomiting activity in BN) in patients with ED. Moreover, this chapter presents recent research on a new carbohydrate marker, the insulinogenic index at 15 minutes, which precisely mirrors eating behaviors in patients with EDs.

Anorexia Nervosa

Anorexia nervosa is a disorder characterized by abnormal eating behavior, weight regulation, and disturbances in attitudes and perceptions toward body weight and shape. Numerous studies have documented abnormalities of physical condition associated with acute anorexia nervosa. In terms of nutritional parameters, McClain et al. evaluated serum and urinary zinc values in patients with anorexia nervosa before and after refeeding, revealing that urinary zinc excretion markedly increased after nutritional rehabilitation [23]. Rock et al. examined the relationship between vitamin status and clinical conditions in patients with anorexia nervosa at admission to a treatment program. They found that thiamin, riboflavin and vitamin B-6 status were normal after refeeding [24]. Moyano et al.'s examination of plasma total-homocysteine, a marker of folate and cobalamin status, in patients with anorexia nervosa revealed that plasma total-homocysteine concentrations significantly increased before refeeding and abnormalities in these values were completely corrected after nutritional rehabilitation [25].

With respect to other biological parameters, Vaisman et al. found that superoxide production by polymorphonuclear cells is correlated with duration of the refeeding period and rate of weight gain [26]. Nova et al. reported that duration of illness and time at which appropriate treatment is achieved were closely associated with alteration of the helper/cytotoxic T cell ratio [27]. Pascal et al. detected high concentrations of sex hormone binding globulin before refeeding, which were normalized after refeeding [28]. Popovic et al. revealed that inhibin B concentrations, a product of the gonads, decreased before weight restoration and increased after refeeding [29].

The results of these previous repeat studies following long-term weight recovery suggest that abnormalities in physical condition relevant to malnutrition are common in acute AN patients, but return to normal with dietary intervention or nutritional rehabilitation. In addition to the above research, a vast literature has shown abnormalities in carbohydrate metabolism in acute and recovered anorexia nervosa. Given these results, we explored the relationship between carbohydrate metabolism and weight restoration in anorexia nervosa and discuss our findings below.

Review of the Literature Concerning Carbohydrate Metabolism and Weight Restoration

Baseline Glucose Concentrations

Anorexia nervosa has been found to exhibit low fasting plasma glucose concentrations of less than 70 mg/dl in the acute phase [30-38]. Tagami et al. reported that acute AN patients showed low fasting plasma glucose concentrations (71.4 mg/dl), but presented normal levels (80.6 mg/dl) after weight restoration [39]. Similarly, Brown et al. also reported that fasting glucose concentrations normalized (90.5 mg/dl) after weight restoration [40].

Baseline Insulin Concentrations

Fasting plasma insulin concentrations have been reported to be typically low or in the lower part of the normal range (between 3.8 and 12 μU/ml) in acute AN patients [30-32, 34, 36-38, 41-43]. In terms of C-peptide, Kobayashi et al. reported that C-peptide secretion was decreased in acute anorexia nervosa [44]; however, other research found that AN patients exhibited similar corresponding plasma C-peptide concentrations when compared to controls [42]. Tagami et al. reported that AN patients showed increases in fasting insulin concentrations after weight restoration (before: 4.9 μU/ml; after: 10.4 μU/ml) [39]; similar findings have also been reported by Crisp et al. and Kalucy et al. [45, 46]. Conversely, other work reported that fasting insulin concentrations were lower than those of healthy control subjects even after weight restoration (4.7 to 7.6 μU/ml) [40, 47].

Insulin Sensitivity and Insulin Resistance

Insulin sensitivity and insulin resistance in anorexia nervosa have been addressed by several investigators. Castillo et al. and Letiexhe et al. used a glucose clamp technique and observed that insulin sensitivity was unchanged in acute AN patients compared to healthy controls [48]. In contrast, Zuniga-Guajardo et al. reported that indices of insulin sensitivity were higher in acute AN patients than controls [38]. Moreover, Kiriike et al. used an insulin clamp technique and observed varying results of insulin sensitivity in acute AN patients [49]. Wachslicht-Rodbard et al. reported elevated insulin binding to erythrocytes in acute AN patients, and suggested increased insulin sensitivity in anorexia nervosa [43]. Zuniga-Guajardo et al. reported that increased insulin sensitivity normalized in AN patients after weight restoration [38]. Moreover, Wachslicht-Rodbard et al. reported that, with increased food intake and weight restoration, the increased insulin binding activity returned to normal, suggesting that this increased insulin sensitivity normalized in AN patients after weight restoration [43].

Glucose Tolerance Test

Abnormalities in carbohydrate metabolism during oral glucose tolerance tests (OGTT) in patients with anorexia nervosa have been well documented. In the acute phase, AN patients showed varying glucose and insulin responses to the OGTT [30, 31, 33, 36, 37, 41, 45, 50-56]. During the OGTT in acute AN patients the glucose response patterns observed were normal type, impaired glucose tolerance type, diabetes mellitus type, and flat type. Impaired glucose tolerance and diabetic response patterns of carbohydrate metabolism in AN patients have also been well documented from the earliest studies, with these responses frequently observed in acute AN patients. Delayed gastric emptying, beta-cell dysfunction, insulin resistance, and impaired neuroendocrine metabolism are reported to be correlated with these responders [30, 36, 37, 54, 57-59], and have been reported to be reversible after weight restoration [33, 41, 45, 54]. Some researchers found that AN patients with severe weight loss also frequently have flat type glucose responses during the OGTT [30, 31, 51, 54, 56]. Prolonged starvation and gastrointestinal dysfunction appear to be associated with these responders in AN [30, 54, 58, 60, 61]. Although Frankel et al. reported that flat type glucose responses were not completely normalized after weight restoration [51], Kanis et al. and Nozaki et al. indicated that these responses normalized after the patients began refeeding [31, 54]. In terms of insulin response patterns to the OGTT, previous research revealed normal type [31, 45, 54], delayed type [31, 45, 54, 55, 62] or low type [54, 63-65] insulin response patterns in acute AN patients. Several researchers have confirmed that these abnormal responses were reversible after weight restoration [31, 51, 54].

Mixed Meal Test

In addition to oral glucose tolerance tests, some researchers examined the effects of mixed meals on carbohydrate metabolism in AN patients [40, 66-68]. In acute AN patients, insulin responses to the test meal were varied and included reduced, normal or increased insulin responses [66, 68]; However, abnormalities in carbohydrate and insulin responses typically normalized after refeeding [66, 68, 69]. Brown et al. reported that glucose responses to the meals in the recovered AN group were similar to those in healthy controls, though the insulin responses to the meal were blunted and apparently delayed compared to controls [40, 67].

Free Fatty Acid (FFA), Growth Hormone (GH) and Cortisol

Several variables such as FFA, GH and cortisol play an important role in the regulation of carbohydrate metabolism. Free fatty acid counter-regulates insulin action, and GH and cortisol have counter-regulatory effects promoting gluconeogenesis and lypolysis. In acute AN patients, FFA levels were reported to be normal or elevated [41, 48, 70]. Changes in FFA concentrations before and after weight restoration were evaluated in several studies. Pirke et al. reported reduced FFA concentrations after weight restoration, although Casper et al. indicated increased FFA concentrations even after refeeding. With respect to GH and cortisol, most research has shown that both fasting plasma GH and cortisol concentrations were increased in acute AN patients [33, 52, 55, 65]. Changes in these variables before and after weight restoration were also evaluated, and several researchers confirmed the normalization of these variables after refeeding [31, 33, 52].

Repeat studies following long-term weight recovery suggest that the metabolic abnormalities frequently seen in acute AN, especially in terms of carbohydrate metabolism, are for the most part elicited by under-nutrition and weight loss, and are reversible after weight restoration. Previous literature suggests the interesting hypothesis that carbohydrate metabolism may be a mirror of weight maintenance; therefore, it is believed that carbohydrate metabolism is a good marker of nutritional status in patients with AN. Although the carbohydrate variables investigated in previous research might be a possible marker of the progress of refeeding in anorexia nervosa, few studies examined the effects of these parameters on treatment-responsiveness in AN patients.

A review of the literature follows a description of our study in which nutritional progress in patients with anorexia nervosa was assessed from the perspective of carbohydrate metabolism during the OGTT. We detected a new carbohydrate marker of nutritional progress, the insulinogenic index at 15 minutes.

Insulinogenic Index at 15 Minutes as a Marker of Refeeding Progress in Anorexia Nervosa

As shown in *Figure 1* [71], we reported a female patient with anorexia nervosa who showed a sharp rise in serum insulin concentrations during the very early phase (15 minutes after glucose loading) of the OGTT, when the patient's daily energy intake was rapidly increased. The results of this case suggested that alterations in eating behaviors might influence early phase carbohydrate metabolism during the OGTT in AN patients; thus, early phase carbohydrate metabolism could be a better marker of nutritional status in these patients.

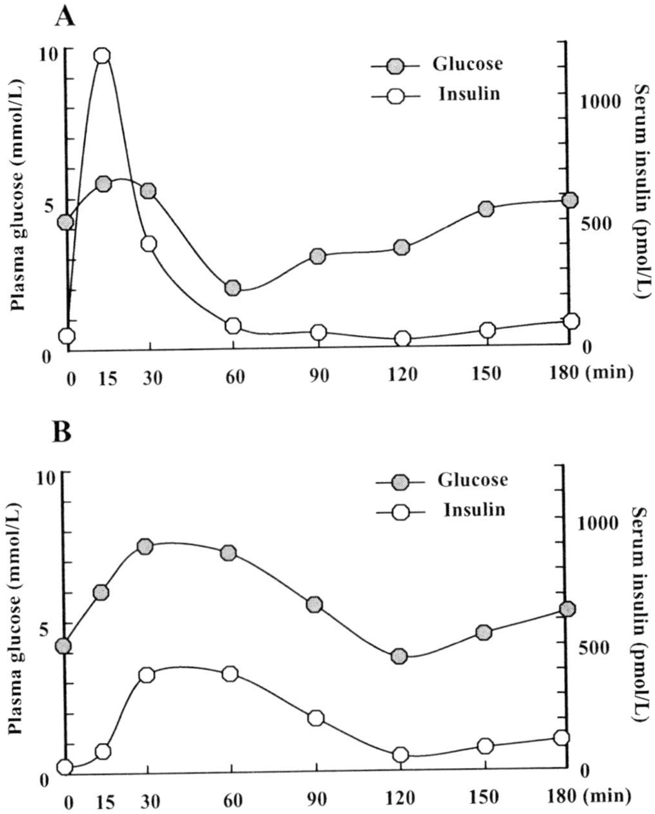

Figure 1. Glucose and insulin response curves during oral glucose tolerance test A)7thday after admission.B)70thday after admission. Source: From YasuharaD et al. *IntJ Eat Disord*2003;34:273-7.

The hypothesis of our previous study was that patients with AN who gain sufficient weight during nutritional rehabilitation might show an increased response of insulin secretion, especially during the early phase of the OGTT [8], as early phase insulin secretion is influenced by the initial increase in blood glucose concentrations and gut hormones after glucose load [72, 73]. In order to determine the relationship between early phase carbohydrate metabolism during the OGTT and the progress of refeeding during nutritional rehabilitation, 48 AN inpatients (25 AN - restrictive type and 23 AN - bulimic type) underwent the OGTT with additional blood sampling at 15 minutes after glucose load. In addition, repeated OGTT was conducted when energy intake reached 1600 kcal/d. Thirteen non-anorectic volunteers were also studied. To evaluate early phase carbohydrate metabolism, we calculated the insulinogenic index at 15 minutes ($II_{15\ min}$) after glucose load, in addition to other carbohydrate variables (e.g., insulin area under the curve, homeostasis model assessment for insulin resistance and $II_{30\ min}$).

$II_{15min} = 0.0077 \times [insulin_{15min} (pmol/L) - insulin_{0min} (pmol/L)] / [blood\ glucose_{15min} (mmol/L) - blood\ glucose_{0min} (mmol/L)]$

Participants were divided into good (≥ 0.5 kg/week) and poor responders (< 0.5 kg/week) based on weekly changes in body weight after patients' daily energy intake reached 1600 kcal/d. Results indicated that $II_{15\ min}$ values for good responders were significantly higher than those for poor responders in both AN subtypes and controls (**Figure 2**), and other variables could not differentiate the responders. This study suggested that the response of very early phase insulin secretion during the OGTT increased in AN patients who responded well to the refeeding program, and implied that the II_{15min} value was an important marker for assessing the progress of nutritional rehabilitation in both AN subtypes, despite significant differences between them in restoration of nutritional status (74). This study also extended the literature on AN by demonstrating that carbohydrate metabolism during the OGTT is correlated not only with under-nutrition before weight restoration but also with the progress of refeeding during nutritional rehabilitation in anorexia nervosa [30, 31, 33, 36, 37, 41, 45, 50-56].

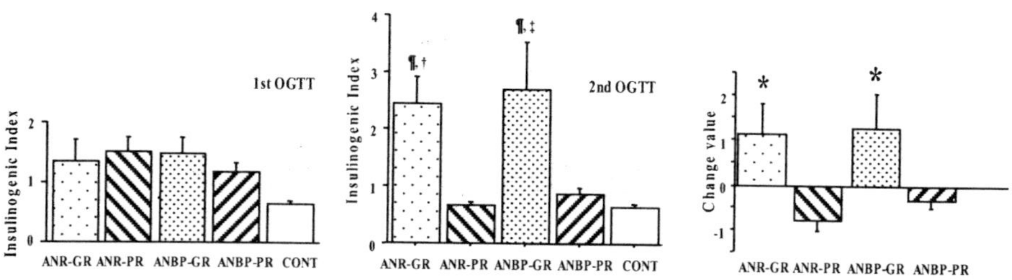

Source: From Yasuhara D et al. Am J Clin Nutr 2003;77:292-9.

Figure 2. Mean(±SE) II15 min values of the first (before refeeding) and second (during refeeding) oral-glucose-tolerance test in patients with anorexia nervosa restricting type who were good responders to treatment (ANR-GR; n = 14), patients with anorexia nervosa restricting type who were poor responders to treatment (ANR-PR; n = 11), patients with anorexia nervosa binge eating–purging type who were good responders to treatment (ANBP-GR; n = 11); patients with anorexia nervosa binge eating–purging type who were poor responders to treatment (ANBP-PR; n = 12), and control subjects (CONT; n = 13). The change value is the difference in the II15 min value between the first and second test. There were no significant differences in the II15 min value on the first test (P = 0.092), but there were significant differences on the second (P = 0.0005). Significantly different from control subjects, P < 0.005. †Significantly different from ANR-PR patients, P < 0.005. ‡Significantly different from ANBP-PR patients, P < 0.005. Two-factor ANOVA showed significant main effects of progress during treatment for the change values (*P = 0.023), but no significant main effects of AN subgroup (P = 0.52) and no progress during treatment–by–AN subgroup interactions (P = 0.72).

Future Research of Markers of Eating Behavior in Anorexia Nervosa

The II_{15min} values appear to precisely mirror nutritional progress in anorexia nervosa and are likely regulated by multiple factors that modify carbohydrate metabolism, including gastrointestinal function [57, 66, 75]and pancreatic beta-cell function [44, 76, 77]. In particular, we considered that neuroendocrine parameters were noteworthy, as Miyawaki et al. reported that a study in gastric inhibitory polypeptide receptor homozygous deficient mice showed impaired insulin secretion early (15 minutes) after glucose load [78]. Therefore, we consider that future research examining the relationships between these parameters and eating behaviors are needed to elucidate the mechanism of the II_{15min} values in anorexia nervosa.

Changes in neuroendocrine parameters before and after refeeding were examined in patients with AN. With regard to anorexigenic hormones, Abell et al. and Geracioti et al. reported normal fasting and post-meal cholecystokinin (CCK) concentrations in AN [66, 79], whereas other researchers observed elevated fasting and post-meal CCK concentrations [80-83], and some researchers confirmed that fasting and post-meal CCK concentrations were normalized after weight gain [66, 82]. Cerebrospinal fluid (CSF) and plasma peptide YY (PYY) concentrations were found to be normal in patients with AN, but the relationship between PYY changes and weight restoration was not examined [84]. In terms of orexigenic hormones, Kaye et al. and Baranowska et al. found that CSF neuropeptide Y (NPY) were increased in acute AN patients [84, 85], whereas plasma NPY were normal or decreased [86]. These abnormalities also normalized in AN patients after weight restoration [84, 85].

Furthermore, recent studies have examined changes in ghrelin and leptin before and after refeeding in anorexia nervosa. With regard to the anorexigenic hormone leptin, plasma leptin levels were low in acute AN patients [35, 86-89], however, decreases in this parameter normalized after weight restoration [40, 84]. In contrast, Balligand et al. reported that this parameter did not respond to short-term refeeding in anorexia nervosa [87]. In terms of the orexigenic hormone ghrelin, plasma ghrelin concentrations in acute AN patients were significantly elevated compared with those of healthy controls [36, 37, 53, 90, 91]. Since ghrelin concentrations returned to normal after partial weight recovery, researchers suggest that ghrelin is a good marker of nutritional status in anorexia nervosa [90, 92]. The results of previous AN research on neuroendocrine parameters showed that abnormalities in acute AN were normalized after weight restoration, suggesting that these parameters might play an important role in abnormal eating behaviors (e.g., severe energy restriction) in anorexia nervosa. Inui et al. addressed that AN patients presented unbalanced shift of feeding-regulatory circuitry (i.e., excess of both orexigenic and anorexigenic signalling), which leaded to a failure of the adaptive feeding response in acute AN patients [93], and therefore, future research examining the relationships between neuroendocrine parameters and eating behaviors may be an important step for determining more useful biologic markers of nutritional status as well as for understanding the core psychopathology of this disorder.

Bulimia Nervosa

In bulimia nervosa, patients follow a chaotic eating behavior pattern, with periods of altered body weight maintenance, including severe energy restriction or binge eating, and compensatory vomiting. Numerous studies have documented abnormalities in physical condition relevant to these abnormal eating behaviors in bulimia nervosa, and specifically, several reports have revealed biological markers of weight maintenance or vomiting activity. Previous studies have addressed that serum/urine electrolytes and serum amylase concentrations were a possible marker of vomiting activity. Several studies have reported serum electrolyte disturbances, such as hypokalemia, hyponatremia, hypochloremia, and metabolic alkalosis in active BN patients [13, 14, 22, 94, 95]. In addition, Greenfeld et al. and

Crow et al. suggested that hypokalemia was closely associated with bulimic behaviors. Moreover, Crow et al. recently examined urine electrolytes in active BN subjects, finding that the ratio of urine sodium to urine chloride was related to bulimic behaviors [12] In terms of serum amylase concentrations, several studies reported elevated serum amylase concentrations in active BN [15-18, 20, 96]. Specifically, some researchers revealed that serum levels of salivary-type amylase were closely associated with vomiting activity in this disorder [16, 20, 96].

Previous studies have documented total serum cholesterol [94, 97-100], thyroid status [70, 101, 102] and vitamin status [24, 103] as biological markers of weight maintenance. Several researchers have reported that total serum cholesterol concentrations were elevated in active BN patients and were normalized after treatment [94, 98, 99] They also suggested that the elevation in serum cholesterol may reflect the excessive dietary intake of cholesterol during binge episodes. With regard to thyroid status, Pirke et al. and Kiyohara et al. reported that active BN patients exhibit decreased T3 (triiodothyronine) and T4 (thyroxine) concentrations, and Pirke et al. suggested that these abnormalities were associated with energy restriction in this disorder [70, 101]. In terms of vitamin status, Rock et al. and Mira et al. both found riboflavin and vitamin B-6 deficiency in patients with active BN, and confirmed that vitamin status is normalized after treatment [24, 103].

In addition to the above research on biological markers of eating behaviors in bulimia nervosa, previous research has revealed a close relationship between carbohydrate metabolism and eating behaviors in active BN patients. Therefore, we explored the relationship between carbohydrate metabolism and abnormal eating behaviors (i.e., altered body weight maintenance and compensatory vomiting activity) in patients with bulimia nervosa.

Review of the Literature Concerning Carbohydrate Metabolism, Weight Maintenance and Vomiting Activity

Baseline Glucose Concentrations

In patients with bulimia nervosa, fasting plasma glucose concentrations have been reported to be normal [77, 104-112] or low [70, 113] compared to healthy controls. Some researchers have suggested that fasting plasma glucose concentrations were normalized after abnormal eating behaviors were normalized [97].

Baseline Insulin Concentrations

Fasting plasma insulin concentrations have been reported to vary between normal [39, 77, 104-106, 108-111, 113, 114], elevated [115, 116] and decreased levels [111]. In terms of the relationship between eating behaviors and carbohydrate metabolism in BN patients, Johnson et al. reported that BN patients showed a reduction in both insulin and glucose concentrations after vomiting activity [114], and other researchers showed that plasma insulin concentrations increased after binges [115-117]. These authors suggested that intermittent food deprivation instigated a hyperinsulinemic response to binge eating as a metabolic defense against starvation.

Insulin Sensitivity and Insulin Resistance

Several investigators have examined insulin sensitivity in bulimia nervosa. Using the euglycemic insulin clamp technique, Kiriike et al. found that insulin sensitivity was decreased in BN patients [49]. In contrast, Raphael et al. used an intravenous insulin tolerance test and reported no difference in insulin sensitivity between BN patients and healthy controls [110]. Moreover, Taniguchi et al. used a modified frequently sampled intravenous glucose tolerance test and found similar results; no significant difference was observed in insulin sensitivity between BN patients and healthy controls [111]. However, relationships between insulin sensitivity and eating behaviors were not investigated in these studies.

Glucose Tolerance Test

Glucose and insulin responses to the OGTT were examined in several studies on BN [77, 104, 107, 111, 114, 116]. In most research, normal glucose and insulin response curves were elicited [77, 104, 111]; therefore, the investigators suggested that, considering body weight maintenance and adequate nutrition, patients with bulimia nervosa possess normal glucose tolerance after oral glucose load. In contrast, Mitchell et al. reported varying types of glucose and insulin response curves on the OGTT, such as flat type and impaired type glucose response curves [107]. Similarly, Russell et al. reported that patients with unstable weight who binged and vomited frequently had blunted insulin responses, patients with stable weight who infrequently binged and vomited had exaggerated insulin response patterns, and responses were normal in successfully treated patients. The authors suggested that the exaggerated insulin response was associated with a physiological adaptation to intermittent starvation, and that the blunted insulin response was related to constant nutritional deprivation in severely ill BN patients [116].

Mixed Meal Test

The effects of mixed meals on carbohydrate metabolism in BN patients were examined by several researchers [21, 106, 108, 112, 114, 115]. Although plasma glucose responses to test meals were similar in BN subjects and healthy controls, insulin responses were elevated [70, 115] or normal [21, 106, 108, 112, 114] in BN subjects. Elevated insulin responses to test meals were frequently observed in BN patients with unstable eating behaviors, and some researchers suggested that these responses represented a metabolic reaction to the intermittent starvation in this disorder [70, 115]. Moreover, in terms of the relationship between vomiting activity and carbohydrate metabolism, Johnson et al. reported that BN patients showed a reduction in both insulin and glucose concentrations after vomiting the test meals, and they suggested that the hypoglycemia resulting from vomiting activity appeared to play an important role in the continuation of repeated binge/purge episodes [114].

FFA, GH And Cortisol

Previous BN research has examined changes in metabolism of FFA, cortisol and GH, which are known to be involved in glucose metabolism and are sensitive to stress and starvation [104]. In terms of FFA, elevated or normal baseline FFA concentrations were observed, suggesting that high FFA was associated with starvation in BN patients who vomited regularly [70, 104]. Bulimic patients who vomited regularly also showed normal [104, 118, 119] or elevated [115, 116, 120-122] basal plasma cortisol concentrations. With regard to the relationship between eating behaviors and plasma cortisol levels, BN patients with stable eating behaviors indicated normal cortisol levels [115, 116, 118, 119]. In contrast, BN patients with unstable eating behaviors (e.g., severe energy restriction or frequent vomiting activity) may be similar to AN patients with elevated cortisol levels [115, 116, 121, 122]. Moreover, some researchers have reported that BN patients showed increased cortisol levels during bingeing, and cortisol levels seemed to return to baseline after cessation of bingeing, suggesting that, because BN patients do not have substantial weight loss, it is possible that abnormal eating behaviors (binge eating, vomiting or intermittent starvation) could alter cortisol metabolism [115]. Basal GH levels were reported by several investigators to be elevated [102, 120, 123] or normal in BN patients [104, 115]. Some researchers have reported abnormal GH responses (increased in most studies) after glucose ingestion or binge eating/vomiting, and suggested that the types of food they had eaten or their actual eating pattern influenced their abnormal GH metabolism [107, 115].

The results of previous studies have suggested that metabolic abnormalities, especially carbohydrate metabolism, as frequently seen in BN patients before treatment, were closely associated with the presence of unstable eating habits, and that these abnormalities are reversible once abnormal eating behaviors are normalized. Previous literature implied that further investigations in terms of carbohydrate metabolism and eating behaviors might aid in the clinical assessment of these patients. We believe that carbohydrate metabolism is a good marker of stable eating behaviors in BN patients. However, few studies had examined the effects of both weight maintenance and vomiting activity on carbohydrate or related variables, which made it difficult to assess the stability of eating behavior using previous biological markers.

A review of the literature follows the next study in which we assessed the stability of eating behaviors in BN patients in consideration of carbohydrate metabolism during the OGTT.

Insulinogenic Index at 15 Minutes as a Marker of Stable Eating Behavior in Bulimia Nervosa

The hypothesis of our study [9] was that II_{15min} might be a useful biological marker of stable eating behavior in patients with BN as well as refeeding progress in anorexia nervosa [8]. We considered that weight maintenance, which mirrored patient's bingeing or intermittent starvation, and the frequency of vomiting were of particular importance to assessing the stability of eating behaviors. In order to determine the relationship between II_{15min} values, weight maintenance, and vomiting activity in patients with BN, 48 bulimic inpatients and 14 controls underwent an OGTT on the 7th hospital day. We calculated II_{15min} and other biological markers, including serum amylase and potassium concentrations. During the first week after admission, we monitored the frequency of vomiting and calculated changes in body weight. Patients were divided into 4 subgroups according to the presence of vomiting and weight loss. A two-factor analysis of variance of the II_{15min} values revealed significant main effects for vomiting and body weight change; the II_{15min} values increased with vomiting activity and decreased with weight loss (see *Figure 3*). The II_{15min} values were positively correlated with serum amylase concentrations, body weight change, and frequencies of vomiting. This study demonstrated that the $II_{15\ min}$ values were closely correlated with weight maintenance in patients with BN as well as AN [8]. Furthermore, this index also associated with vomiting activity, suggesting that the very early phase of carbohydrate/insulin metabolism during the OGTT may precisely mirror abnormal eating behaviors in patients with BN.

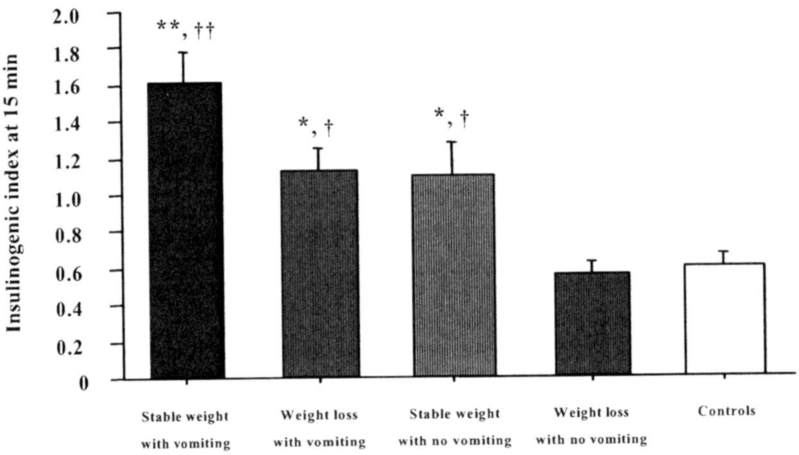

Source: From Yasuhara D et al. *Clin Nutr* 2004;23:711-20.

Figure 3. The II15min values in patients with bulimia nervosa and 14 healthy controls. Patients were classified into 4 groups: 13 patients had weight loss and vomiting, 14 had weight loss and no vomiting, 10 had stable weight (or weight gain) and vomiting, and 11 had stable weight (or weight gain) and no vomiting. Two-factor analysis of variance (vomiting × body weight change) revealed significant main effects for vomiting and body weight change ($P < 0.001$ for both), and no significant interaction between vomiting and body weight change ($P = 0.86$). * $P < 0.005$ vs controls. † $P < 0.005$ vs patients with weight loss and no vomiting ** $P < 0.0001$ vs controls. †† $P < 0.0001$ vs patients with weight loss and no vomiting.

FUTURE RESEARCH OF MARKERS OF EATING BEHAVIORS IN BULIMIA NERVOSA

The $II_{15\ min}$ values appeared to mirror stability of eating behaviors in bulimia nervosa and are likely regulated by multiple factors including gastrointestinal mobility [75], pancreatic B-cell function [77], gut hormones and other neuroendocrine parameters; thus further studies examining the relationships between these parameters, especially neuroendocrine parameters, and eating behaviors are necessary to elucidate the mechanism of the $II_{15\ min}$ values in bulimia nervosa.

With regard to anorexigenic hormones, baseline CCK concentrations were reported to be normal in BN patients [83, 124], whereas CCK responses to a test meal were impaired before treatment [81, 124]. In terms of PYY, CSF PYY levels were normal in patients with chronic bingeing and vomiting and elevated in patients abstinent from bingeing and vomiting [84, 85, 125]. Kaye et al. suggested that abnormally elevated CNS PYY activity in the abstinent state may contribute to a persistent drive in feeding behavior and the resumption of bingeing behaviors [85]. With regard to orexigenic hormones, BN patients before treatment showed high [88] or normal [106] plasma NPY concentrations. After eating behaviors were stabilized, Gendall reported that CSF NPY was normal [84].

Moreover, recent studies examined ghrelin and leptin metabolism from the perspective of eating behaviors in bulimia nervosa. Previous studies reported varying results of normal, decreased and increased levels of anorexigenic hormone leptin in BN [21, 39, 88, 89, 126-129]. Some researchers have reported that plasma leptin concentrations were reduced in BN with long disease duration and a high severity of bingeing and vomiting [128]. In terms of orexigenic hormone ghrelin, several authors have reported that BN patients with bingeing and vomiting exhibit elevated baseline ghrelin levels [106, 130]. Kojima et al. showed reduced ghrelin suppression after a meal and suggested that this finding may contribute to the impaired satiety and binge eating in BN patients [106]. In contrast, Monteleone et al. reported that preprandial plasma ghrelin concentrations were normal and the ghrelin response to food consumption is blunted in symptomatic BN patients; moreover, no significant correlations were identified between plasma ghrelin values and the frequency of binge/vomiting suggesting that altered ghrelin response to food ingestion may be involved in the prolongation of meal and binge eating [108, 131]. The results of previous BN studies suggest that neuroendocrine parameters play an important role in bingeing/vomiting cycles in bulimia nervosa. Moreover, neuroendocrine parameters appear closely correlated with carbohydrate metabolism [132, 133]; therefore, future research examining the relationships between neuroendocrine parameters and abnormal eating behaviors is necessary for elucidating the mechanism of the II_{15min} values as well as determining more useful biologic markers of stable eating behaviors in bulimia nervosa.

CONCLUSION

As the extensive literature suggests, close relationships exist between carbohydrate metabolism and abnormal eating behaviors in patients with EDs. Previous studies on AN have shown various changes in carbohydrate metabolism in the fasting state, and after the ingestion of glucose and test meals; however, these abnormalities were reversible after weight restoration. Moreover, previous BN studies have also revealed a close relationship between abnormalities in carbohydrate metabolism and the presence of unstable eating habits (e.g., weight maintenance and vomiting activity). Although biological parameters relevant to carbohydrate metabolism may be useful for assessing patients' clinical conditions, only a limited number of studies have investigated this issue. Recently, the authors detected a new carbohydrate marker, the insulinogenic index at 15 minutes, which precisely mirrors abnormal eating behaviors (i.e., weight restoration in AN and body weight maintenance and vomiting activity in BN) in patients with EDs. However, the regulatory factors of this index are as yet unclear. This parameter may be influenced by many bio-behavioral, neuroendocrine and nutritional factors. Thus, future research, regarding neuroendocrine parameters regulating satiety and feeding in particular, is necessary for determining more useful biological markers of clinical status as well as elucidating the mechanism of the $II_{15\ min}$ values in anorexia and bulimia nervosa.

References

[1] Hall RC, Hoffman RS, Beresford TP, Wooley B, Hall AK, Kubasak L. Physical illness encountered in patients with eating disorders. *Psychosomatics* 1989;30(2):174-91.

[2] Fairburn CG, Beglin SJ. Studies of the epidemiology of bulimia nervosa. *Am J Psychiatry* 1990;147(4):401-8.

[3] Fairburn CG, Harrison PJ. Eating disorders. *Lancet* 2003;361(9355):407-16.

[4] Steinhausen HC. The outcome of anorexia nervosa in the 20th century. *Am J Psychiatry* 2002;159(8):1284-93.

[5] Zipfel S, Lowe B, Reas DL, Deter HC, Herzog W. Long-term prognosis in anorexia nervosa: lessons from a 21-year follow-up study. *Lancet* 2000;355(9205):721-2.

[6] Beumont PJ, Russell JD, Touyz SW. Treatment of anorexia nervosa. *Lancet* 1993;341(8861):1635-40.

[7] Danziger Y, Carel CA, Tyano S, Mimouni M. Is psychotherapy mandatory during the acute refeeding period in the treatment of anorexia nervosa? *J Adolesc Health Care* 1989;10(4):328-31.

[8] Yasuhara D, Naruo T, Nagai N, Tanaka M, Muranaga T, Nozoe S. Insulinogenic index at 15 min as a marker of nutritional rehabilitation in anorexia nervosa. *Am J Clin Nutr* 2003;77(2):292-9.

[9] Yasuhara D, Tatebe Y, Nakayama T, Muranaga T, Nozoe S, Naruo T. Insulinogenic index at 15 min as a marker of stable eating behavior in bulimia nervosa. *Clin Nutr* 2004;23(4):711-20.

[10] Arden MR, Budow L, Bunnell DW, Nussbaum MP, Shenker IR, Jacobson MS. Alkaline urine is associated with eating disorders. *Am J Dis Child* 1991;145(1):28-30.

[11] Caregaro L, Favaro A, Santonastaso P, et al. Insulin-like growth factor 1 (IGF-1), a nutritional marker in patients with eating disorders. *Clin Nutr* 2001;20(3):251-7.

[12] Crow SJ, Rosenberg ME, Mitchell JE, Thuras P. Urine electrolytes as markers of bulimia nervosa. *Int J Eat Disord* 2001;30(3):279-87.

[13] Crow SJ, Salisbury JJ, Crosby RD, Mitchell JE. Serum electrolytes as markers of vomiting in bulimia nervosa. *Int J Eat Disord* 1997;21(1):95-8.

[14] Greenfeld D, Mickley D, Quinlan DM, Roloff P. Hypokalemia in outpatients with eating disorders. *Am J Psychiatry* 1995;152(1):60-3.

[15] Gwirtsman HE, Kaye WH, George DT, Carosella NW, Greene RC, Jimerson DC. Hyperamylasemia and its relationship to binge-purge episodes: development of a clinically relevant laboratory test. *J Clin Psychiatry* 1989;50(6):196-204.

[16] Humphries LL, Adams LJ, Eckfeldt JH, Levitt MD, McClain CJ. Hyperamylasemia in patients with eating disorders. *Ann Intern Med* 1987;106(1):50-2.

[17] Kinzl J, Biebl W, Herold M. Significance of vomiting for hyperamylasemia and sialadenosis in patients with eating disorders. *Int J Eat Disord* 1993;13(1):117-24.

[18] Kronvall P, Fahy TA, Isaksson A, Theander S, Russell GF. The clinical relevance of salivary amylase monitoring in bulimia nervosa. *Biol Psychiatry* 1992;32(2):156-63.

[19] Marcos A, Varela P, Toro O, Nova E, Lopez-Vidriero I, Morande G. Evaluation of nutritional status by immunologic assessment in bulimia nervosa: influence of body mass index and vomiting episodes. *Am J Clin Nutr* 1997;66(2):491S-7S.

[20] Mitchell JE, Pyle RL, Eckert ED, Hatsukami D, Lentz R. Electrolyte and other physiological abnormalities in patients with bulimia. *Psychol Med* 1983;13(2):273-8.

[21] Monteleone P, Bortolotti F, Fabrazzo M, La Rocca A, Fuschino A, Maj M. Plamsa leptin response to acute fasting and refeeding in untreated women with bulimia nervosa. *J Clin Endocrinol Metab* 2000;85(7):2499-503.

[22] Pyle RL, Mitchell JE, Eckert ED. Bulimia: a report of 34 cases. *J Clin Psychiatry* 1981;42(2):60-4.

[23] McClain CJ, Stuart MA, Vivian B, et al. Zinc status before and after zinc supplementation of eating disorder patients. *J Am Coll Nutr* 1992;11(6):694-700.

[24] Rock CL, Vasantharajan S. Vitamin status of eating disorder patients: relationship to clinical indices and effect of treatment. *Int J Eat Disord* 1995;18(3):257-62.

[25] Moyano D, Vilaseca MA, Artuch R, Valls C, Lambruschini N. Plasma total-homocysteine in anorexia nervosa. *Eur J Clin Nutr* 1998;52(3):172-5.

[26] Vaisman N, Tabachnik E, Hahn T, Voet H, Guy N. Superoxide production during refeeding in patients with anorexia nervosa. *Metabolism* 1992;41(10):1097-9.

[27] Nova E, Samartin S, Gomez S, Morande G, Marcos A. The adaptive response of the immune system to the particular malnutrition of eating disorders. *Eur J Clin Nutr* 2002;56 Suppl 3:S34-7.

[28] Pascal N, Amouzou EK, Sanni A, et al. Serum concentrations of sex hormone binding globulin are elevated in kwashiorkor and anorexia nervosa but not in marasmus. *Am J Clin Nutr* 2002;76(1):239-44.

[29] Popovic V, Djurovic M, Cetkovic A, et al. Inhibin B: a potential marker of gonadal activity in patients with anorexia nervosa during weight recovery. *J Clin Endocrinol Metab* 2004;89(4):1838-43.

[30] Gniuli D, Liverani E, Capristo E, Greco AV, Mingrone G. Blunted glucose metabolism in anorexia nervosa. *Metabolism* 2001;50(8):876-81.

[31] Kanis JA, Brown P, Fitzpatrick K, et al. Anorexia nervosa: a clinical, psychiatric, and laboratory study. I. Clinical and laboratory investigation. *Q J Med* 1974;43(170):321-38.

[32] Mecklenburg RS, Loriaux DL, Thompson RH, Andersen AE, Lipsett MB. Hypothalamic dysfunction in patients with anorexia nervosa. *Medicine* (Baltimore) 1974;53(2):147-59.

[33] Casper RC, Davis JM. On the course of anorexia nervosa. *Am J Psychiatry* 1977;134(9):974-8.

[34] Landon J, Greenwood FC, Stamp TC, Wynn V. The plasma sugar, free fatty acid, cortisol, and growth hormone response to insulin, and the comparison of this procedure

with other tests of pituitary and adrenal function. II. In patients with hypothalamic or pituitary dysfunction or anorexia nervosa. *J Clin Invest* 1966;45(4):437-49.

[35] Pannacciulli N, Vettor R, Milan G, et al. Anorexia nervosa is characterized by increased adiponectin plasma levels and reduced nonoxidative glucose metabolism. *J Clin Endocrinol Metab* 2003;88(4):1748-52.

[36] Tanaka M, Naruo T, Yasuhara D, et al. Fasting plasma ghrelin levels in subtypes of anorexia nervosa. *Psychoneuroendocrinology* 2003;28(7):829-35.

[37] Tanaka M, Tatebe Y, Nakahara T, et al. Eating pattern and the effect of oral glucose on ghrelin and insulin secretion in patients with anorexia nervosa. *Clin Endocrinol (Oxf)* 2003;59(5):574-9.

[38] Zuniga-Guajardo S, Garfinkel PE, Zinman B. Changes in insulin sensitivity and clearance in anorexia nervosa. *Metabolism* 1986;35(12):1096-100.

[39] Tagami T, Satoh N, Usui T, Yamada K, Shimatsu A, Kuzuya H. Adiponectin in anorexia nervosa and bulimia nervosa. J Clin Endocrinol *Metab* 2004;89(4):1833-7.

[40] Brown NW, Ward A, Surwit R, et al. Evidence for metabolic and endocrine abnormalities in subjects recovered from anorexia nervosa. *Metabolism* 2003;52(3):296-302.

[41] Casper RC, Pandey G, Jaspan JB, Rubenstein AH. Eating attitudes and glucose tolerance in anorexia nervosa patients at 8-year followup compared to control subjects. *Psychiatry Res* 1988;25(3):283-99.

[42] Letiexhe MR, Scheen AJ, Lefebvre PJ. Plasma leptin levels, insulin secretion, clearance and action on glucose metabolism in anorexia nervosa. *Eat Weight Disord* 1997;2(2):79-86.

[43] Wachslicht-Rodbard H, Gross HA, Rodbard D, Ebert MH, Roth J. Increased insulin binding to erythrocytes in anorexia nervosa: restoration to normal with refeeding. *N Engl J Med* 1979;300(16):882-7.

[44] Kobayashi N, Tamai H, Takii M, Matsubayashi S, Nakagawa T. Pancreatic B-cell functioning after intravenous glucagon administration in anorexia nervosa. *Acta Psychiatr Scand* 1992;85(1):6-10.

[45] Crisp AH, Fenton GW, Scotton L. The electroencephalogram in anorexia nervosa. *Electroencephalogr Clin Neurophysiol* 1967;23(5):490.

[46] Kalucy RS, Crisp AH, Chard T, McNeilly A, Chen CN, Lacey JH. Nocturnal hormonal profiles in massive obesity, anorexia nervosa and normal females. *J Psychosom Res* 1976;20(6):595-604.

[47] Valevski A, Fridberg G, Gil-Ad I, Laron Z, Weizman A. Neuroendocrinological response to standardized mixed meal in female anorectic patients during active and refeeding phases. *J Pediatr Endocrinol Metab* 2000;13(2):195-9.

[48] Castillo M, Scheen A, Lefebvre PJ, Luyckx AS. Insulin-stimulated glucose disposal is not increased in anorexia nervosa. *J Clin Endocrinol Metab* 1985;60(2):311-4.

[49] Kiriike N, Nishiwaki S, Nagata T, et al. Insulin sensitivity in patients with anorexia nervosa and bulimia. *Acta Psychiatr Scand* 1990;81(3):236-9.

[50] Danowski TS, Livstone E, Gonzales AR, Jung Y, Khurana RC. Fractional and partial hypopituitarism in anorexia nervosa. *Hormones* 1972;3(2):105-18.

[51] Frankel RJ, Jenkins JS. Hypothalamic-pituitary function in anorexia nervosa. *Acta Endocrinol (Copenh)* 1975;78(2):209-21.

[52] Garfinkel PE, Brown GM, Stancer HC, Moldofsky H. Hypothalamic-pituitary function in anorexia nervosa. *Arch Gen Psychiatry* 1975;32(6):739-44.

[53] Nakai Y, Hosoda H, Nin K, et al. Plasma levels of active form of ghrelin during oral glucose tolerance test in patients with anorexia nervosa. *Eur J Endocrinol* 2003;149(1):R1-3.

[54] Nozaki T, Tamai H, Matsubayashi S, Komaki G, Kobayashi N, Nakagawa T. Insulin response to intravenous glucose in patients with anorexia nervosa showing low insulin response to oral glucose. *J Clin Endocrinol Metab* 1994;79(1):217-22.

[55] VanderLaan WP, Parker DC, Rossman LG, VanderLaan EF. Implications of growth hormone release in sleep. *Metabolism* 1970;19(10):891-7.

[56] Warren MP, Vande Wiele RL. Clinical and metabolic features of anorexia nervosa. *Am J Obstet Gynecol* 1973;117(3):435-49.

[57] Dubois A, Gross HA, Ebert MH, Castell DO. Altered gastric emptying and secretion in primary anorexia nervosa. *Gastroenterology* 1979;77(2):319-23.

[58] Scheen AJ, Castillo M, Lefebvre PJ. Insulin sensitivity in anorexia nervosa: a mirror image of obesity? *Diabetes Metab Rev* 1988;4(7):681-90.

[59] Inui A, Uemoto M, Seki W, et al. Rebound hypoglycaemia after intravenous glucose in anorexia nervosa. *Lancet* 1996;347(8997):323-4.

[60] de Zwaan M, Aslam Z, Mitchell JE. Research on energy expenditure in individuals with eating disorders: a review. *Int J Eat Disord* 2002;32(2):127-34.

[61] Russell J, Baur LA, Beumont PJ, et al. Altered energy metabolism in anorexia nervosa. *Psychoneuroendocrinology* 2001;26(1):51-63.

[62] Crisp AH. Some aspects of the evolution, presentation and follow-up of anorexia nervosa. *Proc R Soc Med* 1965;58(10):814-20.

[63] Kumai M, Tamai H, Fujii S, Nakagawa T, Aoki TT. Glucagon secretion in anorexia nervosa. *Am J Clin Nutr* 1988;47(2):239-42.

[64] Nishimura N, Suehiro F, Mitani H, et al. [Endocrine function before and after treatment in patients with anorexia nervosa (author's transl)]. *Nippon Naibunpi Gakkai Zasshi* 1979;55(3):171-82.

[65] Stephan F, Schlienger JL, Blickle JF, de Laharpe F. [Hormonal adaptation to chronic self-starvation in patients with anorexia nervosa (author's transl)]. *Nouv Presse Med* 1982;11(14):1055-8.

[66] Abell TL, Malagelada JR, Lucas AR, et al. Gastric electromechanical and neurohormonal function in anorexia nervosa. *Gastroenterology* 1987;93(5):958-65.

[67] Brown NW, Treasure JL, Campbell IC. Evidence for long-term pancreatic damage caused by laxative abuse in subjects recovered from anorexia nervosa. *Int J Eat Disord* 2001;29(2):236-8.

[68] Schweiger U, Warnhoff M, Pahl J, Pirke KM. Effects of carbohydrate and protein meals on plasma large neutral amino acids, glucose, and insulin plasma levels of anorectic patients. *Metabolism* 1986;35(10):938-43.

[69] Ploog DW, Pirke KM. Psychobiology of anorexia nervosa. *Psychol Med* 1987;17(4):843-59.

[70] Pirke KM, Pahl J, Schweiger U, Warnhoff M. Metabolic and endocrine indices of starvation in bulimia: a comparison with anorexia nervosa. *Psychiatry Res* 1985;15(1):33-9.

[71] Yasuhara D, Deguchi D, Tsutsui J, Nagai N, Nozoe S, Naruo T. A characteristic reactive hypoglycemia induced by rapid change of eating behavior in anorexia nervosa: a case report. *Int J Eat Disord* 2003;34(2):273-7.

[72] Curry DL, Bennett LL, Grodsky GM. Dynamics of insulin secretion by the perfused rat pancreas. *Endocrinology* 1968;83(3):572-84.

[73] Porte D, Jr., Pupo AA. Insulin responses to glucose: evidence for a two pool system in man. *J Clin Invest* 1969;48(12):2309-19.

[74] Kaye WH, Gwirtsman HE, Obarzanek E, George T, Jimerson DC, Ebert MH. Caloric intake necessary for weight maintenance in anorexia nervosa: nonbulimics require greater caloric intake than bulimics. *Am J Clin Nutr* 1986;44(4):435-43.

[75] Kamal N, Chami T, Andersen A, Rosell FA, Schuster MM, Whitehead WE. Delayed gastrointestinal transit times in anorexia nervosa and bulimia nervosa. *Gastroenterology* 1991;101(5):1320-4.

[76] Creutzfeldt W. The incretin concept today. *Diabetologia* 1979;16(2):75-85.

[77] Kobayashi N, Tamai H, Uehata S, et al. Pancreatic abnormalities in patients with eating disorders. *Psychosom Med* 1988;50(6):607-14.

[78] Miyawaki K, Yamada Y, Yano H, et al. Glucose intolerance caused by a defect in the entero-insular axis: a study in gastric inhibitory polypeptide receptor knockout mice. *Proc Natl Acad Sci U S A* 1999;96(26):14843-7.

[79] Geracioti TD, Jr., Liddle RA, Altemus M, Demitrack MA, Gold PW. Regulation of appetite and cholecystokinin secretion in anorexia nervosa. *Am J Psychiatry* 1992;149(7):958-61.

[80] Harty RF, Pearson PH, Solomon TE, McGuigan JE. Cholecystokinin, vasoactive intestinal peptide and peptide histidine methionine responses to feeding in anorexia nervosa. *Regul Pept* 1991;36(1):141-50.

[81] Phillipp E, Pirke KM, Kellner MB, Krieg JC. Disturbed cholecystokinin secretion in patients with eating disorders. *Life Sci* 1991;48(25):2443-50.

[82] Tamai H, Takemura J, Kobayashi N, Matsubayashi S, Matsukura S, Nakagawa T. Changes in plasma cholecystokinin concentrations after oral glucose tolerance test in anorexia nervosa before and after therapy. *Metabolism* 1993;42(5):581-4.

[83] Fujimoto S, Inui A, Kiyota N, et al. Increased cholecystokinin and pancreatic polypeptide responses to a fat-rich meal in patients with restrictive but not bulimic anorexia nervosa. *Biol Psychiatry* 1997;41(10):1068-70.

[84] Gendall KA, Kaye WH, Altemus M, McConaha CW, La Via MC. Leptin, neuropeptide Y, and peptide YY in long-term recovered eating disorder patients. *Biol Psychiatry* 1999;46(2):292-9.

[85] Kaye WH, Berrettini W, Gwirtsman H, George DT. Altered cerebrospinal fluid neuropeptide Y and peptide YY immunoreactivity in anorexia and bulimia nervosa. *Arch Gen Psychiatry* 1990;47(6):548-56.

[86] Baranowska B, Wasilewska-Dziubinska E, Radzikowska M, Plonowski A, Roguski K. Neuropeptide Y, galanin, and leptin release in obese women and in women with anorexia nervosa. *Metabolism* 1997;46(12):1384-9.

[87] Balligand JL, Brichard SM, Brichard V, Desager JP, Lambert M. Hypoleptinemia in patients with anorexia nervosa: loss of circadian rhythm and unresponsiveness to short-term refeeding. *Eur J Endocrinol* 1998;138(4):415-20.

[88] Baranowska B, Wolinska-Witort E, Wasilewska-Dziubinska E, Roguski K, Chmielowska M. Plasma leptin, neuropeptide Y (NPY) and galanin concentrations in bulimia nervosa and in anorexia nervosa. *Neuro Endocrinol Lett* 2001;22(5):356-8.
[89] Monteleone P, Di Lieto A, Tortorella A, Longobardi N, Maj M. Circulating leptin in patients with anorexia nervosa, bulimia nervosa or binge-eating disorder: relationship to body weight, eating patterns, psychopathology and endocrine changes. *Psychiatry Res* 2000;94(2):121-9.
[90] Otto B, Cuntz U, Fruehauf E, et al. Weight gain decreases elevated plasma ghrelin concentrations of patients with anorexia nervosa. *Eur J Endocrinol* 2001;145(5):669-73.
[91] Shiiya T, Nakazato M, Mizuta M, et al. Plasma ghrelin levels in lean and obese humans and the effect of glucose on ghrelin secretion. *J Clin Endocrinol Metab* 2002;87(1):240-4.
[92] Soriano-Guillen L, Barrios V, Campos-Barros A, Argente J. Ghrelin levels in obesity and anorexia nervosa: effect of weight reduction or recuperation. *J Pediatr* 2004;144(1):36-42.
[93] Inui A. Eating behavior in anorexia nervosa--an excess of both orexigenic and anorexigenic signalling? *Mol Psychiatry* 2001;6(6):620-4.
[94] Mira M, Stewart PM, Vizzard J, Abraham S. Biochemical abnormalities in anorexia nervosa and bulimia. *Ann Clin Biochem* 1987;24 (Pt 1):29-35.
[95] Palla B, Litt IF. Medical complications of eating disorders in adolescents. *Pediatrics* 1988;81(5):613-23.
[96] Walsh BT, Wong LM, Pesce MA, Hadigan CM, Bodourian SH. Hyperamylasemia in bulimia nervosa. *J Clin Psychiatry* 1990;51(9):373-7.
[97] Gendall KA, Joyce PR, Carter FA, McIntosh VV, Bulik CM. The effect of bulimia nervosa on plasma glucose and lipids. *Physiol Behav* 2002;77(1):99-105.
[98] Halmi K, Fry M. Serum lipids in anorexia nervosa. *Biol Psychiatry* 1974;8(2):159-67.
[99] Sullivan PF, Gendall KA, Bulik CM, Carter FA, Joyce PR. Elevated total cholesterol in bulimia nervosa. *Int J Eat Disord* 1998;23(4):425-32.
[100] Vize CM, Coker S. Hypercholesterolemia in bulimia nervosa. *Int J Eat Disord* 1994;15(3):293-5.
[101] Kiyohara K, Tamai H, Kobayashi N, Nakagawa T. Hypothalamic-pituitary-thyroidal axis alterations in bulimic patients. *Am J Clin Nutr* 1988;47(5):805-9.
[102] Levy AB, Dixon KN, Malarkey WB. Pituitary response to TRH in bulimia. *Biol Psychiatry* 1988;23(5):476-84.
[103] Mira M, Stewart PM, Abraham SF. Vitamin and trace element status of women with disordered eating. *Am J Clin Nutr* 1989;50(5):940-4.
[104] Casper RC, Pandy GN, Jaspan JB, Rubenstein AH. Hormone and metabolite plasma levels after oral glucose in bulimia and healthy controls. *Biol Psychiatry* 1988;24(6):663-74.
[105] Karhunen LJ, Lappalainen RI, Tammela L, Turpeinen AK, Uusitupa MI. Subjective and physiological cephalic phase responses to food in obese binge-eating women. *Int J Eat Disord* 1997;21(4):321-8.
[106] Kojima S, Nakahara T, Nagai N, et al. Altered ghrelin and peptide YY responses to meals in bulimia nervosa. *Clin Endocrinol* (Oxf) 2005;62(1):74-8.

[107] Mitchell JE, Bantle JP. Metabolic and endocrine investigations in women of normal weight with the bulimia syndrome. *Biol Psychiatry* 1983;18(3):355-65.

[108] Monteleone P, Martiadis V, Fabrazzo M, Serritella C, Maj M. Ghrelin and leptin responses to food ingestion in bulimia nervosa: implications for binge-eating and compensatory behaviours. *Psychol Med* 2003;33(8):1387-94.

[109] Moyer A, Rodin J, Cummings N. Cephalic phase insulin release in bulimia. *Int J Eat Disord* 1993;14(3):331-9.

[110] Raphael FJ, Rodin DA, Peattie A, et al. Ovarian morphology and insulin sensitivity in women with bulimia nervosa. *Clin Endocrinol* (Oxf) 1995;43(4):451-5.

[111] Taniguchi A, Nakai Y, Fukushima M, et al. Intravenous glucose tolerance test-derived glucose effectiveness in bulimia nervosa. *Metabolism* 1997;46(5):484-6.

[112] Weingarten HP, Hendler R, Rodin J. Metabolism and endocrine secretion in response to a test meal in normal-weight bulimic women. *Psychosom Med* 1988;50(3):273-85.

[113] Devlin MJ, Walsh BT, Kral JG, Heymsfield SB, Pi-Sunyer FX, Dantzic S. Metabolic abnormalities in bulimia nervosa. *Arch Gen Psychiatry* 1990;47(2):144-8.

[114] Johnson WG, Jarrell MP, Chupurdia KM, Williamson DA. Repeated binge/purge cycles in bulimia nervosa: role of glucose and insulin. *Int J Eat Disord* 1994;15(4):331-41.

[115] Kaye WH, Gwirtsman HE, George DT. The effect of bingeing and vomiting on hormonal secretion. *Biol Psychiatry* 1989;25(6):768-80.

[116] Russell J, Hooper M, Hunt G. Insulin response in bulimia nervosa as a marker of nutritional depletion. *Int J Eat Disord* 1996;20(3):307-13.

[117] Taylor AE, Hubbard J, Anderson EJ. Impact of binge eating on metabolic and leptin dynamics in normal young women. *J Clin Endocrinol Metab* 1999;84(2):428-34.

[118] Gold PW, Gwirtsman H, Avgerinos PC, et al. Abnormal hypothalamic-pituitary-adrenal function in anorexia nervosa. Pathophysiologic mechanisms in underweight and weight-corrected patients. *N Engl J Med* 1986;314(21):1335-42.

[119] Walsh BT, Roose SP, Katz JL, et al. Hypothalamic-pituitary-adrenal-cortical activity in anorexia nervosa and bulimia. *Psychoneuroendocrinology* 1987;12(2):131-40.

[120] Coiro V, Volpi R, Marchesi C, et al. Abnormal growth hormone and cortisol, but not thyroid-stimulating hormone, responses to an intravenous glucose tolerance test in normal-weight, bulimic women. *Psychoneuroendocrinology* 1992;17(6):639-45.

[121] Kennedy SH, Garfinkel PE, Parienti V, Costa D, Brown GM. Changes in melatonin levels but not cortisol levels are associated with depression in patients with eating disorders. *Arch Gen Psychiatry* 1989;46(1):73-8.

[122] Mortola JF, Rasmussen DD, Yen SS. Alterations of the adrenocorticotropin-cortisol axis in normal weight bulimic women: evidence for a central mechanism. *J Clin Endocrinol Metab* 1989;68(3):517-22.

[123] Kiriike N, Nishiwaki S, Izumiya Y, Maeda Y, Kawakita Y. Thyrotropin, prolactin, and growth hormone responses to thyrotropin-releasing hormone in anorexia nervosa and bulimia. *Biol Psychiatry* 1987;22(2):167-76.

[124] Geracioti TD, Jr., Liddle RA. Impaired cholecystokinin secretion in bulimia nervosa. *N Engl J Med* 1988;319(11):683-8.

[125] Berrettini WH, Kaye WH, Gwirtsman H, Allbright A. Cerebrospinal fluid peptide YY immunoreactivity in eating disorders. *Neuropsychobiology* 1988;19(3):121-4.

[126] Brewerton TD, Lesem MD, Kennedy A, Garvey WT. Reduced plasma leptin concentrations in bulimia nervosa. *Psychoneuroendocrinology* 2000;25(7):649-58.

[127] Jimerson DC, Mantzoros C, Wolfe BE, Metzger ED. Decreased serum leptin in bulimia nervosa. *J Clin Endocrinol Metab* 2000;85(12):4511-4.

[128] Monteleone P, Fabrazzo M, Tortorella A, Fuschino A, Maj M. Opposite modifications in circulating leptin and soluble leptin receptor across the eating disorder spectrum. *Mol Psychiatry* 2002;7(6):641-6.

[129] Nakai Y, Hamagaki S, Takagi R, Taniguchi A, Kurimoto F. Plasma concentrations of tumor necrosis factor-alpha (TNF-alpha) and soluble TNF receptors in patients with bulimia nervosa. *Clin Endocrinol* (Oxf) 2000;53(3):383-8.

[130] Tanaka M, Naruo T, Muranaga T, et al. Increased fasting plasma ghrelin levels in patients with bulimia nervosa. *Eur J Endocrinol* 2002;146(6):R1-3.

[131] Monteleone P, Fabrazzo M, Tortorella A, Martiadis V, Serritella C, Maj M. Circulating ghrelin is decreased in non-obese and obese women with binge eating disorder as well as in obese non-binge eating women, but not in patients with bulimia nervosa. *Psychoneuroendocrinology* 2005;30(3):243-50.

[132] Salehi A, Dornonville de la Cour C, Hakanson R, Lundquist I. Effects of ghrelin on insulin and glucagon secretion: a study of isolated pancreatic islets and intact mice. *Regul Pept* 2004;118(3):143-50.

[133] Seufert J, Kieffer TJ, Habener JF. Leptin inhibits insulin gene transcription and reverses hyperinsulinemia in leptin-deficient ob/ob mice. *Proc Natl Acad Sci U S A* 1999;96(2):674-9.

In: Eating Disorders and Weight Loss Research
Editor: Jerome S. Rubin, pp. 127-162
ISBN 1-60021-334-0

Chapter 6

DIETS FOR WEIGHT REDUCTION IN OBESITY, CARDIOVASCULAR DISEASE, HYPERTENSION AND THE METABOLIC SYNDROME: THE GUIDELINES, THE POPULAR DIETS AND THE SPECIAL DIETARY INTERVENTIONS

Annie Ferland and Paul Poirier[1]
Institut universitaire de cardiologie et de pneumologie,
Hôpital Laval, Université Laval, Sainte-Foy, Québec, Canada

INTRODUCTION

It is well recognized that the prevalence of metabolic abnormalities found in the presence of obesity is increasing within our sedentary population. In fact, obesity is a growing epidemic that is primarily due to environmental influences. There has been a rapid increase in obesity over the past 30 years in North America, whereas the recent prevalence estimations from self-reported data in Canada indicated that 15 % of the adult population is obese and 33 % is classified in the overweight category, while in the US nearly 1/3 of adults are obese, corresponding to almost 20 % of the US population [1-3]. This highlights the importance of environmental factors and lifestyle choices since obesity cannot be totally explained by genetic factors alone [4]. Unfortunately, sedentary lifestyle and increased energy intake predispose to high fat and high calorie food choices, and refined diet seems to be adopted by an increasing proportion of our population. This is leading to weight gain, positive energy balance, obesity and health-related complications. Thus, "at risk" obesity (abdominal obesity) is an important cause of metabolic complications, such as cardiovascular disease (CVD), type 2 diabetes, hypertension, and the metabolic syndrome (MetS) [5-7]. Indeed, the American Heart Association (AHA) has classified obesity as a modifiable risk factor for coronary heart

[1] Corresponding author:Paul Poirier MD, PhD, FRCPC, FACC,Institut universitaire de cardiologie et de pneumologie ,Hôpital Laval,2725 Chemin Sainte-Foy ,Sainte-Foy, Québec, Canada,G1V 4G5,Telephone: 418-656-4767,Fax: 418-656-4562,E-mail:Paul.Poirier@crhl.ulaval.ca

disease (CHD) [8]. A variety of therapies may help to reduce the incidence of obesity and the MetS, including diet, physical exercise, and pharmacological treatments. Weight loss is an essential component in the management of the metabolic complications of obesity as well as the MetS itself. Low-fat diets have been advocated for weight loss for many years. However, some popular diets such as the very low-carbohydrate (ketogenic) diets have challenged the effectiveness of conventional low-fat diets, partly because of there rapid efficiency in contrast to the continuing increased prevalence of obesity despite reductions of fat intake. Thus, several authors have compared the effectiveness of various weight loss approaches, such as those proposed by the official guidelines, to the "popular" diets (as Atkins, Ornish, The Zone, South Beach diet, Weight Watchers) in the management of obesity and its related complications. Although, there is a need to perform well designed clinical trials showing long-term safety and efficacy of low-carbohydrate diets, several studies have showed effective short-term weight loss and improved metabolic characteristics of the MetS compared to low-fat diets. The major targets of intervention for proper treatment of the epidemic of obesity remain weight loss and active lifestyle. Even if different types of diet or diet/exercise combinations can produce weight loss; if this treatment is stopped, weight is regained. The current review underlines the clinical and the experimental evidence of the different dietary approaches for weight loss regarding obesity treatment and related metabolic complications. Despite numerous researches, there is still controversy regarding the optimal macronutrient content, and we also overview the issue of carbohydrate restriction versus fat restriction on weight loss and weight control in order to achieve effective weight loss and better health. Indeed, modest weight reduction (5 % to 10 % of body weight) can decrease total cholesterol, improve glucose tolerance and decrease blood pressure in overweight and type 2 diabetic patients [6;9-12]. This review also discusses the consequences of obesity management on the MetS, which represents a cluster of several specific metabolic abnormalities recognized to increase CVD, type 2 diabetes and cardiovascular mortality [6;7;13]. Considering that recent prospective studies show that obesity seems to be the central component of the MetS [5;6], and epidemiological studies have showed that these high-risk individuals have a three-fold increment in CVD and cardiovascular mortality, weight loss is recommended as a first-line therapy [7;14;15]. We also briefly discuss the role of several dietary interventions, which can lower CHD risk and improve lipid profile.

The Metabolic Syndrome

The MetS is a cluster of cardiovascular risk factors that may be attributable to insulin resistance. In 1999, the World Health Organisation (WHO) was the first to attempt to achieve an internationally recognized definition of the MetS [16]. They included either glucose intolerance or insulin resistance as an essential component of the definition [16]. Subsequently in 2001, the National Cholesterol Education Program Adult Treatment Panel III (NCEP-ATP III) has formulated specific criteria for clinical identification of the MetS [7], followed by the International Diabetes Federation and the American Heart Association/National Heart, Lung, and Blood Institute (AHA/NHLBI) in 2005 [6;17]. Actually, it is estimated that 47 millions US adults meet the NCEP-ATP III criteria for the MetS [18]. The MetS is defined by at least three of the five following risk factors: 1) abdominal obesity, 2) elevated triglycerides (TG), 3) low HDL-cholesterol level, 4) elevated fasting glucose and, 5) elevated blood pressure [6;7]. However, this definition differs from the WHO criteria's in terms of insulin resistance and the AHA/NHLBI definition in regard to glucose intolerance (6;7;16). Recently, the International Diabetes Federation (IDF) has established a new definition for the MetS, highlighting ethnic specific values for waist circumference and areas where more research is needed [17]. MetS is linked to an altered insulin efficiency, which can be related to genetic predisposition in light of excess weight and physical inactivity. Table 1 shows the criteria's of the MetS proposed by the NCEP-ATP III, WHO, the IFD and the AHA/NHLBI. Although there are several other classifications of the MetS, the NCEP-ATP III criteria are those that are commonly used considering their usefulness in clinical practice [6;7;16;17;19].

Table 1. Criteria for identification and diagnosis of the metabolic syndrome proposed by the National Cholesterol Education Program Adult Treatment Panel III (NCEP-ATP III), the World Health Organisation (WHO) the American Heart Association/ National Heart, Lung, and Blood Institute (AHA/NHLBI) and the International Diabetes Federation (IDF)

Risk factors	**NCEP-ATP III** *At least 3 or more of these risk determinants are present*	**WHO** *Impared glucose tolerance, insulin resistance or diabetes AND ≥ 2 risk determinants*	**AHA & NHLBI** *At least 3 or more of these risk determinants are present*	**IDF** *Presence of abdominal obesity and 2 of these 4 risk determinants*
Abdominal obesity	Waist circumference Women : > 88 cm Men : > 102 cm	Waist-to-hip ratio: Women : > 0.85 Men : > 0.90 and/or BMI > 30 kg/m^2	Waist circumference Women : > 88 cm Men : > 102 cm	Waist circumference (different values for different ethnics) Women: > 80 cm caucasians Men: > 94 cm caucasians
HDL-cholesterol	Women : < 1.29 mmol/L Men : < 1.03 mmol/L	Women : < 1.0 mmol/L Men : < 0.9 mmol/L	Women : < 1.29 mmol/L Men : < 1.03 mmol/L	Women : < 1.1 mmol/L Men : < 1.03 mmol/L Or pharmacological treatment
Triglycerides	≥ 1.69 mmol/L	≥ 1.7 mmol/L	≥ 1.69 mmol/L	≥ 1.7 mmol/L or pharmacological treatment
Blood pressure	≥ 130/85 mm Hg	≥ 140/90 mm Hg	≥ 130/85 mm Hg	≥ 130/90 mm Hg or treatment or diagnostic of high blood pressure
Fasted glucose	≥ 6.1 mmol/L	Glucose intolerance or diabetes	≥ 5.6 mmol/L	≥ 5.6 mmol/L or diabetes

Adapted from references 6, 7, 16 and 17

The primary clinical approach is weight reduction and increased physical activity with concomitant reduction in LDL-cholesterol levels by dietary and other lifestyle modification and/or use of pharmacological treatment [7]. Of note, the LDL-cholesterol criterion is not a part of the definition of the MetS. The aggressiveness of the lowering cholesterol intervention will depend upon the presence of elevated or very elevated plasma LDL-cholesterol, or the presence of several risk factors of coronary artery disease (CAD) [19]. The second phase of the MetS intervention is the modification of the other risk factors such as blood pressure, triglycerides and HDL-cholesterol levels [7;18]. In summary, major changes in lifestyle are unavoidable and involve: 1) reduction of the dietary contribution in total cholesterol and saturated fat, 2) increased daily physical activity and, 3) achievement of weight control [7].

Considering the global epidemic of obesity and diabetes, it is very likely that the prevalence of the MetS will increase in the North American population during the next decades. According to the estimations of the National Health and 3 or more of the 5 criteria associated to the MetS [18]. Moreover, the prevalence is six-fold greater in a population older than 60 years old compared with young adults from 20 to 29 years old [18]. Each variable associated with the MetS is by itself a risk factor for other diseases including diabetes mellitus and CAD, exposing all this population to multiple cardiovascular complications. Hence, morbidity and mortality are dramatically increased.

Multiple Risk Factors Related to Obesity, Cardiovascular Disease, Type 2 Diabetes and the Metabolic Syndrome

1. Blood Cholesterol and Lipoprotein Profile

Elevated LDL-cholesterol is one of the leading cause of CAD. The American Heart Association (AHA) and the National Cholesterol Education Program (NCEP-ATP III) emphasizes dietary measures to achieve LDL-cholesterol goals, since reduction in LDL-cholesterol levels are associated with reduced CAD risk [7;20]. The food components, which have a major negative impact on LDL-cholesterol, are dietary saturated fatty acids, *trans*-unsaturated fatty acids and cholesterol. Dietary recommendations have emphasized the consumption of monounsaturated and polyusaturated fatty acids, and, to a lesser extent, soluble fibre and soy protein [20]. The NCEP- ATP III report has updated the recommendations for clinical management of high blood cholesterol, considering LDL-cholesterol as the primary target of cholesterol-lowering intervention [7]. Moreover, the recent AHA/NHLBI statement has proposed minor modifications to the NCEP-ATP III criteria by lowering the actual fasting blood glucose target [6]. Assessment of the lipid profile is also a basic constituent of the diagnostic of the MetS. It is recommended to measure lipid profile (total cholesterol, LDL-cholesterol, HDL-cholesterol and TG) in the fasted state every 5 years in adults aged 20 years or older [6;7]. The NCEP-ATP III and the AHA/NHLBI recommendations about the optimal cholesterol target is maintaining total cholesterol below 5.2 mmol/L and raising HDL-cholesterol to the highest extent possible [6;7]. It is generally advised to modifie cholesterol target in function of the presence of one or more risk factors such as cigarette smoking, high blood pressure (≥140/90 mm Hg), low HDL-cholesterol (<1,03 mmol/L), familial history of early CAD (aged ≤ 45 years for men and ≤ 55 years for women) [6;7]. In the absence of risk factors or the presence of only one risk factor, one is permitted to target a LDL-cholesterol below 4.14 mmol/L. The presence of two or more risk factors suggests targeting a LDL-cholesterol level below 3.36 mmol/L. The ultimate categorie considered very high risk is the one associated with the presence of CVD or diabetes. These patients should attain the lowest range of LDL-cholesterol (<2,59 mmol/L). Of note, sustained weight loss is an important issue regarding LDL-cholesterol management in some individuals [20].

2. Abdominal Obesity

It is now well known that abdominal fat distribution is strongly correlated with an increase in morbidity [5]. In fact, central distribution of fat is clearly related to metabolic complications of obesity such as insulin resistance, diabetes, hypertension or CAD in addition to the overall level of obesity by itself [21;22]. Moreover, abdominal obesity is an important feature of the MetS. Indeed, it is clearly demonstrated that a high level of visceral fat is associated to a high level of small LDL-cholesterol particles and development of impaired glucose tolerance in obese subjects [21;23;24]. Since not all obese people should be considered at high risk of CAD, it is important for the clinician to use simple and effective tools to identify the obese "at risk" [25;26]. Clinicians may use simple non-invasive measurements to assess body fat and estimate easily abdominal obesity.

The AHA and the National Institute of Health (NIH) have adopted the Quetelet-Kaup index, or body mass index (BMI), as an indicator to measure adiposity and classify people as normal, overweight or obese [9]. The Canadian definition to classify people as overweight or obese is also defined by BMI, in accordance to the World Health Organization (WHO) guidelines and Health Canada [27;28]. BMI is defined as weight in kilograms divided by height in meters squared (kg/m^2). Obesity is defined by a BMI >30 kg/m^2 and overweight by a BMI between 25 and 29.9 kg/m^2 [9;27;28]. Waist circumference is probably a more useful tool that all clinician should use to evaluate abdominal fat during weight loss treatment. Although BMI and waist circumference are interrelated, increased waist circumference can be a better predictor of disease risk in adults who are categorized as normal or overweight in terms of BMI [9;26]. In accordance to the BMI and waist circumference definition, adults aged 18 years or more with a BMI between 25 and 34.9 kg/m^2 and a waist circumference of ≥ 102 cm for men and ≥ 88 cm for women have an increased risk for cardiovascular co-morbidity [9]. Considering that waist circumference is closely correlated to visceral adipose tissue and metabolic complications, simultaneous measurement of simple variables such as waist circumference and fasting plasma TG levels have also been suggested to be used as an inexpensive screening tool to identify men and women with high CAD risk [22;29]. Recently, the INTERHEART study has reported that classification of obesity measured by BMI is weaker than the waist-to-hip ratio in order to evaluate the risk of myocardial infarction worldwide [5]. This ratio, strongly related to visceral fat, was the best anthropometric predictor of myocardial infarction in both sexes, regardless of the presence of diabetes, dyslipidemia or hypertension, and in smokers and non-smokers [5]. Moreover, Yusuf et al have suggested that the use of waist-to-hip ratio as an obesity index instead of BMI may increase threefold the risk for myocardial infarction [5]. Abdominal obesity can also worsen the prognosis of patients with CAD. These patients have a 23 % increase risk of myocardial infarction and a 38 % increase risk of heart failure [26]. The factors related to obesity are complex and multifactorial, and lifestyle intervention should play a predominant role [7;9;26;30]. Table 1 present the classification of normal weight, overweight and obesity according to the BMI and waist circumference.

3. Hypertension

The preponderance of high blood pressure is an important problem, while being a modifiable risk factor of CVD. About 43 millions individuals in United States have high blood pressure and only 47 % maintain optimal blood pressure [31]. Reducing weight by lifestyle modifications is a non-pharmacological recommended approach to reduce hypertension. Daily consumption of alcohol and sodium must be reduced since they can impact negatively on optimal blood pressure [32]. The 2005 Canadian Hypertension Education Program have recommended blood pressure target below 140/90 mm Hg in the presence of non-complicated hypertension or systolic hypertension, <130/80 mm Hg in the presence of diabetes and renal dysfunction and <125/75 mm Hg when hypertension is associated to proteinuria (>1g /24h) [33]. Presently, there are no clearly recommended target values in the presence of the MetS. However, values >130/85 mm Hg (NCEP-ATP III and AHA/NHBLI) and 140/90 mm Hg (WHO) are considered abnormal in the MetS classification [6;7;13;16].

Reducing Cardiovascular Disease by Dietary Practices: the Conventional Nutritional Approaches

Changes in deleterious lifestyle habits are considered the most efficient and the less expensive way to reduce cardiovascular risk. The INTERHEART study have identified nine modifiable risk factors; lipoprotein profile, smoking, hypertension, diabetes, abdominal obesity, psychosocial factors, consumption of fruits and vegetables, alcohol intake, and regular physical activity, which predicts 90% of myocardial infarction worldwide in both sexes [34]. Since numerous patients with hypertension, CVD or MetS are overweight or obese and present high-risk waist circumference [35-37], weight loss should be the first line therapy prescribed by health professionals [8;20] This approach may improve insulin sensitivity and influence positively each metabolic abnormality (i.e. hypertension, diabetes, lipid disorder or preexisting CVD). Improved insulin sensibility (30-60 %) associated with substantial weight loss will be of benefit until there is weight regain [38]. Several methods and strategies are available, and it is important to target the right approach in order to achieve and maintain a healthy body weight. The awareness of foods and overall eating pattern must be emphasized.

The AHA has established guidelines for reducing the risk of CVD by dietary and other lifestyle practices [20;39]. The energy balance should be maintained by matching the intake of energy to overall energy expenditure to achieve a healthy body weight. Patients must include a variety of fruits, vegetables, whole grains and cereal products, low-fat dairy products, low saturated fat and lean meats while eating adequate amounts of essential nutrients [20]. This eating pattern is essential to prevent or delay the development of obesity, hypertension, CVD, MetS or other health related complications. Portion number and size should be monitored, and consumption of foods with low nutritional quality, high caloric density and refined sugars should be limited [20]. In general, a relative caloric restriction from 5% to 10% through 6 months is sufficient to reduce several risk factors of heart disease and stroke in people who are overweight or obese with comorbidities, even if optimal weight is not attained [9;19;40]. Increasing level of physical activity is also essential to achieve cardiovascular fitness and energy imbalance to induce weight reduction. Moreover, physical activity reduces the risk of high blood pressure, heart disease and diabetes [33;41]. Sedentary individuals are encouraged to practice 30 to 45 minutes of moderate level of physical activities and subsequently increase these activities to 60 minutes on most if not all days of the week [6;20;33;41;42].

Caloric restriction is a common approach to create energy imbalance and weight reduction. A diet high in total fat is sometimes associated with excess body weight and high-density food choices [43]. Caloric restriction around 500 to 1000 kcal/day is recommended to achieve weight reduction [9;19;20]. Of importance, the optimal weight loss diet must have adequate nutritional composition to reduce risk factors. Guidelines for weight maintenance and weight reduction from AHA (previously designed Step 1 diet), NCEP-ATP III and the North American Association for the Study of Obesity /National Institute of Health (NAASO/NIH) recommended that total calories should be limited to <30 % as fat to pinduce a weight loss of 0.5 to 1 kg per week. The general element of the majority of existing recommendations is the use of a moderate caloric deficit to achieve a slow and progressive weight loss [6;7;9;20]. Dietary components, which influence directly LDL-cholesterol and promote thrombogenesis are saturated fat, cholesterol and *trans*-fatty acids. To achieve reduction in LDL-cholesterol, saturated fat intake should be limited to <7 % of the total energy intake, cholesterol level to less than 200 mg/day and 2 % to 3 % of total energy from *trans*-fatty acids (AHA nutrition therapy for specific subgroups, previously designed Step 2 diet for higher-risk individuals) [20]. These goals can be achieved by limiting intake of foods high in saturated fat, cholesterol and/or *trans*-fatty acids, such as tropical oils, fatty meats, egg yolks, shellfish, high-fat dairy products and prepared foods containing partially hydrogenated vegetable oils. Saturated fat should be substituted for higher proportion of monounsaturated fat, polyunsaturated fat and carbohydrate (e.g., more than 10% of total calories from polyunsaturated fat, more than 15 % of total from monounsaturated fat and 55% or more of total calories from complexes carbohydrates) [9;20]. Protein should be derived from lean sources of animal protein or plant sources and should provide approximately 15 % of total calories. Multiple evidences have shown that salt intake is directly related to high blood pressure and that lowering salt intake lowers blood pressure [32;44;45]. In fact, reducing sodium intake by 1800 mg per day (which correspond to 2/3 teaspoon of table salt) or achieving an average daily consumption of 2400 mg (1 teaspoon of table salt) is associated with systolic and diastolic blood pressure reductions [32;44;45]. Of note, the average intake of sodium in the United States is approximately 3500 mg per day (1½ teaspoon of table salt) [45]. Reducing sodium intake by choosing foods low in salt and limiting the amount of salt added to food is also an important target. Moreover, alcohol consumption should not exceed more than 2 drinks per day for men and 1 drink per day for women.

The practical guideline for identification, evaluation and treatment of overweight and obesity in adults from the NIH and NAASO recommends low calorie diet (which corresponds to the Step 1 diet from AHA) to induce weight loss in overweight and obese patients [9;20]. In general, diets containing 1000 to 1200 kcal per day should be recommended to most women. More so, diets between 1200 to 1600 kcal per day should be selected for men and for women who weigh 75 kg or more [9].

A more drastic approach for obese individuals presenting numerous risk factors is a very low calorie diet, providing approximately 800 kcal per day [19]. This diet requires special monitoring and supplementation, should be used in very limited circumstances, and under intensive medical supervision [9]. The common use of these diets decreased considerably during the last decades, corresponding to 50 % in the 1960s to 7,7 % in the 1990s (46). Weight reduction is generally more important under very low calorie diets vs. low calorie diets but several clinical trials reported that low calorie diets are as effective as very low calorie diet in producing weight loss after 1 year. On the other hand, significant weight regain is common regarding these diets [47;48]. The use of a very low calorie diet has been associated with significant long-term advantages. Wadden et al have compared weight loss of 49 obese women over one-year, randomly assigned to a low calorie diet (1200 kcal per day) and a very low calorie diet (420 kcal per day, for 16 weeks followed with 1200 kcal per day for 36 weeks) [48]. Women under the very low calorie diet lost significantly more weight through the first 26 weeks. However, they regained more easily their weight through the 26 weeks of the weight maintenance phase. Total weight losses after one year were comparable between the 2 groups, with a mean decrease of 11kg for the very low calorie diet and 12kg for the low calorie diet [48]. More so, the very low calorie diet, as liquid-protein-diet, has been associated with a prolonged QT interval and with sudden death [49]. These complications may be related to vitamin and mineral deficiencies, to a poor quality and/or inadequate quantity of protein consumed per day, to various concomitant drug regimen used by patients or to a prolonged adhesion to this kind of diet [50]. However, under appropriate medical control, no significant change of QT interval was reported [51;52].

Reducing Blood Pressure: The DASH Diet

It is well known that obesity, high sodium intake and alcohol consumption influence arterial blood pressure (BP). Recent evidences have shown that approximately 60 % of American adults have prehypertension or hypertension (53). Moreover, the two major goals of the dietary recommendations in the presence of CVD or the MetS are to lower BP and improve serum lipids. The Dietary Approaches to Stop Hypertension (DASH)-diet is a carbohydrate-rich diet, currently advocated in several scientific dietary reports and guidelines such as the AHA and the NCEP-ATP III, for the prevention and treatment of BP in individuals with and without hypertension [9;20;32;45;54-56]. Table 2 presents the number of serving for each food group between the DASH diet and the Canada's food guide to healthy eating. The DASH trial demonstrated that a diet that emphasized vegetables, fruits and low-fat dairy products, whole grains, poultry, fish and nuts, and a limited amount of red meat, sweets and sugar-containing beverages, a decrease amounts of total fat, saturated fat and cholesterol can substantially lower mean systolic BP from 7.1 mm Hg in people without hypertension to 11.5 mm Hg in people with hypertension [32;44]. The Seventh Report of the Joint National Committee on Prevention, Detection, Evaluation, and Treatment of High Blood Pressure (JNC7) recommends several lifestyle modifications in order to manage hypertension. The major lifestyle modifications which have shown to lower BP include weight reduction which may reduce systolic BP by 5 mm Hg to 20 mm Hg per 10-kg weight loss, adoption of the DASH eating pattern and reducing the daily dietary sodium intake to no more than 100 mmol or 2.4 g sodium or 6 g sodium chloride (one teaspoon of sodium chloride = 2.4 g of sodium) [57]. More so, the alcohol consumption should be limited to no more than 2 drinks in most men and no more than one drink per day in women and lighter-weight individuals (1 drink is equivalent to a 341 mL beer, 150 mL glass of wine and 45 mL of spirituous) [57]. The effects of three different levels of dietary sodium intake in conjunction with the DASH diet or a control diet on 412 participants for 30 consecutive days was studied [45]. The subjects were randomly assigned to eat foods with high levels of sodium (150 mmol/day or 1½ teaspoon of table salt per day with an energy intake of 2100 kcal, reflecting the typical consumption in the United States), intermediate intake (100 mmol/day or 1 teaspoon of table salt per day, reflecting the upper limit of the current JNC7 national recommendations) and low intake (50 mmol/day or ½ teaspoon of table salt per day, below the current recommendation of 100 mmol/day from the DASH diet) [45]. A significant decrease in BP (-11.4 mm Hg and –5.5 mm Hg for the systolic BP and the diastolic BP respectively) were observed in the combined 50 mmol sodium intake/DASH diet intervention group [45].

Table 2. Number of serving for each food group between the DASH diet and Canada's food guide to healthy eating.

	Number of serving Canada's food guide to healthy eating	Number of serving DASH diet
Fruit	5-10 per day	4-5 per day
Vegetables		4-5 per day
Milk products	2-3 per day	2-4 per day
Grain products	5-12 per day	7-8 per day

Adapted from Canada's food guide to healthy eating & Appel LJ et coll. N Engl J Med 336:1117-1124, 1997

The Canadian Hypertension Education Program for the management of Hypertension has proposed recent recommendations [33]. These recommendations include lifestyle and nutritional modifications to prevent and/or treat hypertension such as: 30 to 60 minutes of aerobic exercise per day, achieving and maintaining an ideal body weight and waist circumference, limiting alcohol intake, reducing total fat and cholesterol intake and limiting salt consumption [33]. The European Society of Hypertension and the European Society of Cardiology have also proposed guidelines, which are similar to the DASH, the JNC7 and the Canadian Hypertension Education Program recommendations [58]. Table 3 presents the lifestyle modifications to manage hypertension proposed by the DASH diet, the JNC7, the Canadian Hypertension Education Program and the European Society of Hypertension.

Table 3. Lifestyle modifications to manage hypertension proposed by the Dietary Approaches to Stop Hypertension (DASH)-diet, The Seventh Report of the Joint National Committee on Prevention, Detection, Evaluation, and Treatment of High Blood Pressure (JNC7), The Canadian Hypertension Education Program for the management of hypertension and the European Society of Hypertension/European Society of Cardiology.

	DASH	JNC7	Canadian Hypertension Education Program	European Society of Hypertension
Weight reduction	Maintain ideal body weight	Maintain body weight: 18.5 kg/m^2 to 24.9 kg/m^2 *↓ 5-20 mm Hg systolic BP per 10-kg weight loss*	Maintain body weight: (18.5 kg/m^2 to 24.9 kg/m^2) Waist circumference: < 102 cm for men < 88 cm for women	Weight reduction to maintain ideal body weight
Maximal alcohol intake	2 drinks per day for most men 1 drink per day for women	2 drinks per day for most men 1 drink per day for women	14 drinks per week (2 drinks/day) for most men 9 drinks per week (1.3 drinks/day) for women	20-30 ml alcohol/day for men (30 ml = 2 drinks) 10-20 ml alcohol/day for women (15 ml = 1 drink)
Physical exercise	--	≥ 30 minutes of aerobic exercise most days of the week	30-60 minutes of aerobic exercise 4-7 days per week	30-45 minutes of aerobic exercise 3-4 days per week
Sodium intake	100 mmol or 2.4 g sodium per day (1 teaspoon of table salt)	100 mmol or 2.4 g sodium per day (1 teaspoon of table salt) *↓ 2-8 mm Hg systolic BP*	100 mmol or 2.4 g sodium per day (1 teaspoon of table salt)	80-100 mmol/day or 1.9-2.4 g per day (2/3 – 1 teaspoon of table salt) *↓ BP 4-6 mm Hg*
Total fat	Decrease total fat, saturated fat and cholesterol Consume low-fat dairy products *↓ 7.1-11.5 mm Hg*	Decrease total fat and saturated fat Consume low-fat dairy products *↓ 8-14 mm Hg systolic BP*	Decrease total fat and cholesterol	Decrease total fat and saturated fat
Fruits and vegetables	Emphasized fruits an vegetables	Consume a diet rich in fruits and vegetables	Increase fruits and vegetables	Increase fruist and vegetables

Adapted from references 33, 56, 57 and 58

Lowering saturated fat intake is also an important target in the presence of hypertension and high serum lipids. The Lyon Diet Heart Study proposes a Mediterranean-type diet characterized by a low intake of total and saturated fats, increase intake of ω-3 fatty acids, high intake of fresh fruits, vegetables, whole grain cereals, antioxidants, vitamins, minerals and vegetable proteins [59]. An increase of 1 mm Hg of systolic BP is associated with an increase risk of 1 % to 2% of cardiovascular complications after myocardial infarction [59]. The optimal macronutrient substitutions for saturated fat (carbohydrate, protein or unsaturated fat) were recently evaluated in the OMNIHEART trial [60]. Three different diet interventions were assessed, such as a high-carbohydrate diet (similar to the DASH diet), a diet rich in protein (10 % higher in protein than the 2 other diets) and an unsaturated fat diet (10% higher in unsaturated fat sources such as olive oil, canola and safflower oil). Interestingly, partial substitution of carbohydrate with either protein or monounsaturated fat can further lower BP, improve lipid levels and reduce CVD risk [60].

THE NON CONVENTIONAL NUTRITIONAL APPROACH (POPULAR DIETS)

Insulin sensitivity may be influenced by the total caloric intake and the diet composition. Many conditions such as overweight and abdominal obesity are clearly associated with altered insulin sensitivity. Low physical activity level and genetic factors also contribute to deteriorate several metabolic pathways. Caloric restriction and weight loss have been shown to improve glucose metabolism in glucose intolerant and type 2 diabetic patients [61]. In the presence of type 2 diabetes, a weight loss of about 5 % of the initial weight is sufficient to improve insulin sensitivity, fasted glucose and glycated hemoglobin [10]. Data from the Framingham study have demonstrated that an isolated weight loss in the order of 3 to 7 kg (approximately 5 % to 10 % of the initial weight) results in a 33 % decrease incidence of diabetes. Moreover, a more important weight loss is even more beneficial [62]. Diets with a high proportion of simple sugars and/or fructose, or high in saturated fat may be related to insulin resistance and decreased HDL-cholesterol levels [63;64]. Moreover, the increased activity of the sympathetic nervous system and the renal sodium retention associated with hyperinsulinemia may also contribute to high blood pressure [65].

Considering the alarming increase in the incidence and the prevalence of obesity and diabetes, a large proportion of people experiment popular diets, which promote spectacular weight loss without efforts advocating important changes in carbohydrate and lipid consumption. Many of these diets restrain consumption of carbohydrate and have increased lipid consumption in order to restrict daily caloric consumption and increase satiety. Diets that may influence the postprandial insulin secretion are: glycemic index (GI), the Zone diet, the South Beach diet and the very low carbohydrate diets which induce satiety by increasing ketosis and decreasing gastro-intestinal motility (Atkins) [40]. Three different popular diets will be discussed further;

1. "Average" diet, such as the Mediterranean diet and the Weight Watchers program
2. Low-carbohydrate-diet or GI diet, very-high-protein diet (e.g. GI index, the Montignac diet, and the Zone diet)
3. Very low carbohydrate diet/very-high-protein/fat diet (e.g. Atkins and the South Beach diet);
4. Very-low-fat/Very-high-carbohydrate diet (e.g. Ornish).

"Average" Diet

The Mediterranean Diet

For many years, Mediterranean diet has been associated with beneficial effects related to cardiovascular health, cancer and increased life expectancy [59;66-68]. The increasing interest of this diet resulted from the Seven Countries Study from Keys et al., which demonstrated that traditional Mediterranean diet conferred a decrease mortality rate from CHD principally because of a low saturated fat content [67]. Many definitions characteristic of the Mediterranean diet have been suggested. In fact, the broad geographical region including the 16 countries that border the Mediterranean Sea and the different cultural, ethnic and agricultural production include different dietary practice. The Mediterranean-style diet related to a specific dietary pattern, has been presented in a pyramid by Willett WC et al [69]. The diet is characterized by abundant intakes of fresh fruits and vegetables, whole grain products, monounsaturated fat from olive oil and low-fat dairy product (principally from cheese and yogurt). Traditional Mediterranean diet also incorporates the following components: 1) high monounsaturated-to-saturated fat ratio, 2) moderate alcohol consumption and, 3) low consumption of meat and meat products. Some studies defined differently the daily consumption of meat, suggesting abundant intake of fish and poultry, and a restricted-to-moderated consumption of eggs (zero to 4 eggs per week) [69;70]. There is also a definition in terms of the macronutrients pattern, which supplied 25 % to 30 % of total energy intake from fat, with restricted consumption of saturated fat (<7 % to 8 % from total energy intake). Monounsaturated fats, antioxidants-rich foods (such as cranberries, blueberries or blackberries), high-fiber, and selenium rich foods (such as Brazil nuts, seafood or poultry) are also suggested [69]. A prevention trial performed by De Lorgeril et al has shown the cardioprotective effects of a Mediterranean type diet [68]. They report a 70 % reduction in the recurrence of myocardial infarction and cardiac death following a diet of <35 % of the energy as fat (from rapeseed oil), <10 % of energy as saturated fat, <4 % of the energy as ω-6 fatty acids and >0.6 % of energy as ω-3 fatty acids. The Lyon Diet Heart 4-year follow-up study has compared the traditional Mediterranean diet (increased fruits, vegetables, green legumes, fish, poultry and decreased red meat, pork, and butter) to the conventional diet for weight maintenance and weight reduction as suggested by the AHA (previously designed Step 1 diet) on the reduction of the rate of recurrence after a first myocardial infarction [59]. After 46 months of follow-up, the group following the Mediterranean diet presented a 72 % reduction in cardiac death and non-fatal myocardial infarction. Moreover, the risk of recurrent heart disease was lowered by 56 % [59]. The Mediterranean diet is also associated with beneficial modifications in total cholesterol, apoB concentration and LDL size particle [71-73]. Recently, Esposito K. et al have shown that a 2-year adherence to a Mediterranean-style diet is effective in reducing the prevalence of the MetS and its associated cardiovascular risk [66]. Endothelial function and vascular inflammatory markers were assessed in 180 patients with MetS. Patients in the intervention group have increased total daily consumption of fruits, vegetables, whole grains, nuts, and olive oil in accordance to the Mediterranean style diet. A significant weight loss was observed in the intervention group (-4.0 kg vs. –1.2 kg for the control group), reduced serum hs-CRP levels and inflammatory markers as well as decreased insulin resistance and improved endothelial function were also observed [66]

The Weight Watchers Program

The Weight Watchers program is a low-calorie diet designed to produce a weight loss of up to 0.9 kg per week. This program includes a food plan based on an exchange system list provided by the Weight Watchers corporation which determine point values of common food. The patient's total daily «points» allowance is determined by the current weight. Each "point" is equivalent to approximately 50 calories. The food plan is nutritionally balanced and the activity plan follows the current guidelines. The Weight Watchers program has also a behaviour modification plan for weight control focusing primarily on cognitive restructuring. Participants generally attend a 1-hour weekly group meeting to promote social support, provide written educational material and to weigh oneself weekly. Weight Watchers has sponsored 4 randomized, controlled trialson its program. Heshka et al. have compared the effect of a self-sufficient intervention to the commercial Weight Watchers program on weight loss in 423 overweight/obese men and women (average starting weight of 94.2 kg) [74]. Participant in the Weight Watchers group lost 4.8 kg of their initial weight during the 26 weeks treatment (-1.4 kg for the self-sufficient intervention group). Another study was performed in a cohort of 48 women with a history of breast cancer to prevent adverse prognosis related to obesity [75].

.They were randomly assigned to receive usual care, attend a weekly Weight Watchers group meeting, undergo individual counselling with a dietician, or receive both of the latter 2 interventions. At 1-year, the Weight Watchers group had lost 2.6 kg, those who had individual counselling lost 8.0 kg, those who underwent both interventions lost 9.4 kg and participants who received usual care gained 0.9 kg [75]. Higher weight loss is often achieved in the Weight Watchers groups compared to the standard diet or the control diet, because of the high rate of adherence in these groups, which was partly proportional to the frequency of the counselling approach and the individualized contact [74-76] Lowe et al have evaluated the weight loss maintenance among 1002 participants who had reached their goal weight 1 to 5 years previously. These results suggest a weight regain range between 31.5 % and 76.5 % from the initial weight [77]. Table 4 presents a summary of the main changes in the macronutrient composition of the conventional and the various average diets.

Low-Carbohydrate-Diet (and GI Index Diet)/Very-High-Protein Diet

Low Carbohydrate Diet or Glycemic Index of Food

Although controversial, the GI of foods is still a popular approach for weight loss and has been shown to improve insulin sensitivity in the presence of the MetS [78]. Some international associations have adopted the GI as nutritional therapy for weight management as well as for type 2 diabetes. However, it is not the case of the American Diabetes Association and several other associations in the United States [79]. The WHO and the Food and Agriculture Organisation (FAO) have endorsed, since 1998, the use of the GI of food as an indicator of the impact of a carbohydrate-rich food on blood glucose response and have supported it as an interventional strategy in the treatment of diabetes, in conjunction with information about food composition to guide food choices [80;81]. This committee emphasizes the importance of carbohydrates in human nutrition for the promotion of good health and recommends the consumption of a high-carbohydrate diet (>55 % of total energy).

Moreover, emphasis in carbohydrate-containing foods rich in non-starch polysaccharides with low GI are suggested. Actually, many official and/or suggested dietary guidelines and carbohydrate exchanges lists of food currently used for diabetes management are based on the GI of food in Australia, Canada and South Africa [82;83]. The GI concept is now more commonly used due to its potential for disease prevention related to lifestyle habits. In Australia, certain foods are incorporated in a GI trademark certification program labelling. A symbol is affixed on food labels to help consumers select low-GI foods. The nutritional composition meets the criteria established for a category of particular food. Moreover, the Australian dietary guidelines specifically recommend the consumption of low-GI cereal foods in order to achieve good health.

Table 4. Changes in the macronutrient composition of the conventional and the various average diets

	Moderate fat diets				Average diet	
	AHA Step I Diet (11)	AHA Step II Diet (11)	NCEP-ATPIII Diet (5)	DASH diet (45)	Mediterranean-Style (Lyon Heart study) (55)	Weight Watchers program (124)
Total fat (% kcal)	≤ 30	≤ 30	25 - 30	27	31	27
Saturated fat	8-10	< 7	< 7	6	8	10
Polyunsaturated	> 10	> 10	> 10	8	5	--
ω-6 linoleic acid	--	--	--	--	4	--
ω-9 oleic acid	--	--	--	--	1	--
Monounsaturated	> 15	> 15	> 20	13	13	--
Cholesterol (mg)	300	200	200	150	200	184
Carbohydrate (% kcal)	≥ 55	≥ 55	50-60	55	53	53
Protein (% kcal)	15	15	15	18	16	20
Fiber (g)	20-30	20-30	20-30	> 30	19	15
Sodium (mmol)	100	100	100	< 100	< 100	--
Alcohol (% kcal)	--	--	--	--	6	--

Adapted from references 7, 20, 56, 59, 137

David J. A. Jenkins has proposed the first table of GI of foods in 1981, and has published a list of 51 foods with their respective GI [84]. He has suggested that the proposed GI list may reflect the physiological effect of foods, since different carbohydrate foods with the same macronutrient composition can induce a different glycemic response. Per gram of carbohydrate, foods with a high GI produce a higher peak in postprandial blood glucose and a greater overall blood glucose response during the first 2 hours following the consumption of the carbohydrate-rich food than do foods with a low GI. According to Jenkins, the GI of food calculation is calculated using the area under the positive blood glucose response curve in response to the consumption of 50 g of carbohydrate provided by the proposed food divided by the area under the blood glucose response curve following the consumption of 50 g of carbohydrate provided by the control foods, generally white bread or sucrose [85;86]. Many food factors may influence the measure and the reproducibility of GI: 1) the type and the amount of protein and fat (decreases the blood glucose response), 2) the type and the amount of carbohydrate (ratio of amylose and amylopectin in the selected food) and fibres (fibres reduce the rate of absorption of glucose from the gut), 3) food processing and cooking (rise in blood glucose and insulin following the consumption of cooked as opposed to raw foods, and increase time of cooking is associated with an increase of glycemic response), 4) the ripeness of the food (changes in composition of the fruits as they are ripen can increase the glycemic response) and, 5) food processing (grinding, extruding and flaking can increase glycemic response) [87-89].

It is well documented that the low-GI index can achieve better metabolic and glycemic control in type 2 diabetic individuals [90-95], increase HDL-cholesterol concentration, decrease LDL-cholesterol and triglycerides concentrations [96-98], increase satiety [99-104] and improve insulin sensitivity [78]. Moreover, observational studies have shown that the chronic consumption of a diet with a high glycemic load (GI x dietary carbohydrate content) is independently associated with an increase risk of developing type 2 diabetes and CVD [105-107]. Some studies assume that the quantity and the quality of dietary carbohydrate can play a critical role in the pathogenesis of obesity and the MetS [108-110]. Kopp et al have hypothesized that the current North-American high-glycemic index intake can induce a progressive dysregulation of the pancreatic beta cells, an adaptive hypertrophy of the pancreas resulting in postprandial hyperinsulinemia and insulin resistance, secondary to the chronic high-insulin stimulus in genetically predisposed subjects [110]. Moreover, some studies suggest that postprandial hyperinsulinemia decreases satiety and promotes glucose oxidation to the detriment of free fatty acids through lipolysis inhibition, inducing fat storage [110-112]. Consuming low-GI foods can be an efficient method to reduce daily energy intake and achieve weight control, through the decrease in appetite and the increase of satiety [100;103;113], as well as promoting free fatty acids oxidation [101]. Until now, more than 750 foods have been tested to assess their GI [114]. The low-GI foods include the majority of fruits and vegetables, leguminous and whole wheat bread, whereas high-GI foods include refined cereals products such as white bread, potatoes and rice. In general, when glucose is used as the standard for the GI measure, it is recommended to privilege most of the time food having a low-GI, equal or lower than 55, to consume periodically foods having a GI between 56 and 69 and avoid those which are higher than 70 [114]. However, it is generally agreed that there is a need for long-term clinical trials to establish the clinical relevance and the use of GI in relation to weight regulation, obesity, type 2 diabetes and CVD [115-118].

The Montignac Method

The Montignac Method is a low-GI index/low-fat/high-protein diet, which has been popular in Canada and Europe and was one of the first diets using the GI of foods in daily life. This diet is characterized by a low-GI index (GI < 50), low-fat-high-protein content and emphasis on the quality of food and the physiologic effects on blood glucose response [119]. The Montignac Method also recommends avoiding the combination of high-carbohydrate and high-fat foods in the same meal, unless the GI of carbohydrate foods are below 20 [119;120]. Combining high-carbohydrate/low-GI to high-protein foods and high-protein to high-fat foods in the same meal is also recommended. Food consumption is *ad libidum* until satiety [119;120]. Monounsaturated fat and polyunsaturated fat should be privileged over saturated fat in order ot achieved cardiovascular prevention [120]. Moreover, foods choices should be high in fibres to promote satiety [119]. The short term impact of the Montignac diet compared to the AHA diet for weight maintenance and reduction (Step 1 diet) on the metabolic profile of 12 overweight men has been reported [121]. The Montignac diet has shown to induce a spontaneous 25 % and 35 % decrease of daily energetic intake and plasma TG levels respectively. Moreover, a significant increase in LDL-cholesterol particle diameter and marked decreases in plasma insulin levels were also observed [121].

The South Beach Diet

The South Beach diet has been elaborated by Arthur Agatston, a cardiologist from Miami, who wanted to recommend a way for his heart disease patients to lose weight in a healthy, sustainable way. The South Beach diet emphasizes the "good carbohydrates" (low-GI) and "good fat" (17 % of total caloric intake from monounsaturated fat and 32 % to 14 % from polyunsaturated, varying through the 3 phases of the diet) and lean protein and uses the GI in order to choose the right foods to consume during this weight loss program [122]. It is speculated that the important glycemic response following the consumption of high-GI foods is directly related to weight gain and should be avoided during any kind of weight loss diet. However, most of the nutritional principles and theories regarding this diet are sparsely referenced in the book [122].

Three phases have to be followed through the South Beach diet. The initial phases of the diet consist of 2 phases of 2 weeks duration each and a third phase of 8 weeks for weight maintenance. The first 2 weeks is characterized by higher intake of fat (62 %) and protein (28 %), with a very low intake of carbohydrates (10 %). Not surprisingly, normal size portions should be consumed, and lean meat, fish, eggs, reduced-fat cheese, non-fat yogurt, nuts, and vegetables should be chosen. Bread, rice, potatoes, fruits, alcohol, sweets or every carbohydrate foods should be avoided during this period (2 weeks) to diminish sweetened foods craving. In the second phase, fat intake is decreased to 43 % whereas protein intake is increased to 30 % and carbohydrate intake to 27 %. Finally, during the phase 3, percentages of calories are 39 % from fat, 33 % from protein and 28 % from carbohydrate [122]. The conventional NCEP-ATPIII diet was compared to a isocaloric modified low-carbohydrate/high protein and monounsaturated fat diet (South Beach diet). The investigators found a greater weight loss over 3 months (6.1 kg vs. 3.4 kg for the South Beach compared to the NCEP-ATPIII diet respectively) with no significant amelioration in regard to blood lipid levels between groups [123].

The Zone Diet

The Zone diet is a low-carbohydrate/high protein diet. Percentages of daily total calories are approximately 36 % from carbohydrates, 34 % from protein and 29 % from fat (with 9 % from saturated fat) [124]. The "philosophy" behind the diet from the author Dr Barry Sears asserts that eating the right combination of foods (carbohydrates to protein and fat ratio) leads to decreased hunger, enhanced weight loss and increased energy [125]. The proponent of the Zone Diet suggest enhanced lipolysis through the regulation of glucose and insulin levels which optimize the body's metabolic function [125]. This diet does not prohibit particular foods or food groups. An emphasis is made on carbohydrates from fruits and vegetables sources and monounsaturated fat (such as olive oil, avocado, or almonds). However, high fat (or saturated fat) and high carbohydrates foods such as starches, bread, pasta and some types of fruit should be avoided [124;125]. Moreover, it seems imperative to eat in exact proportion (40/30/30) carbohydrate, protein and fat at each meal to attain the nutritional balance of the diet. A calculation system has been establish, as a equivalent system: it is recommended for a men to consume 4 blocks of carbohydrate, 4 blocks of protein and 4 blocks of fat at each meal and 1 block each of carbohydrate, protein and fat during snacks. The equivalents for women are 3 blocks during the meals and 1 during snacks. One block of protein is equivalent to 7 g (for example, 30 g of low-fat cheese), one block of carbohydrate is equivalent to 9 g (for example, considering the density, 1 block of carbohydrate is equivalent to ¼ cup of black eye peas or 10 cups of lettuce) and 1 block of fat is equivalent to 1.5 g (for example, 1/3 teaspoon of olive oil). Recently, Miyashita et al. have compared the impact of a low calories/low-carbohydrate diet (1000 kcal; 40 % carbohydrate, 25 % protein, and 35 % of fat) to a low calories/high carbohydrate diet (1000 kcal; 65 % carbohydrate, 25 % protein, and 10 % fat) on glucose, lipid metabolism, and on visceral fat accumulation. Twenty-two obese subjects with type 2 diabetes were randomly assigned to take one of these 2 diets for 1 month [126]. Considering that the 2 diets were equivalent in terms of total calories, a similar decrease in body weight and serum glucose levels was observed in both groups. However, an increase in serum HDL-cholesterol and a important decrease of visceral fat was observed in the low-carbohydrate diet group [126].

Actually, the Zone Diet, as all high-protein diets, is not recommended by the AHA in order to achieve weight loss [124]. Increasing protein proportion in the diet usually leads to increase intakes of total fat, saturated fat and cholesterol since the protein content is mainly from animal sources. Moreover, these types of diets can compromise intake of foods that provide essential vitamins and minerals, as well as potentially inducing cardiac, renal, bone and liver abnormalities [124]. The current premise of high-protein diets is interesting since it is related with low insulin levels associated with carbohydrates restrictions, which can play a role in weight regulation by enhancing lipolysis. Although insulin may play a role in weight regulation, protein intake can also stimulate postprandial insulin secretion and can result in either no change or a modest decrease in postprandial glucose levels [127-129]. Insulin may be regulated by several interacting factors, such as a 4-fold greater increase in glucagon secretion in response to a high-protein diet, resulting in a stimulation of gluconeogenesis, glycogenolysis and subsequent increase in circulating glucose concentrations [129]. Visceral obesity is associated with an increase in circulating insulin levels, which is known to acutely inhibit fat mobilization and oxidation. Moreover, these kinds of diets are often rigid and difficult to maintain long term.

Very-Low-Carbohydrate/Very-High-Protein/Fat Diet

The increasing popularity of diets with emphasis on carbohydrates restriction and high-protein intake are a concern in the United States and in Canada because of the lack of scientific evidence to support their claims associated with potential short and long-term adverse impacts on overall health. The popular version of this kind of diet recommends a severe restriction of daily carbohydrate intake to 20 g per day (the Atkins diet or the first phase of the South Beach diet), or approximately 5 % of total energy [130]. This carbohydrate restriction associated with a high-protein and high-fat diet content induces metabolic ketosis and subsequently a rapid weight loss. However, this initial weight loss may be attributed to loss of appetite associated with ketosis and to the diuretic effect of low-carbohydrates intake [131]. Some studies have reported the weight loss efficacy of low-carbohydrates diets regarding lipid profile. The effects of these diets were evaluated in the presence of obesity and/or dyslipidemia and diabetes [132-136]. Yancy et al have observed in 120 dyslipidemic obese subjects with a mean body weight of 96.8 kg, a two-fold weight loss decrease in the low-carbohydrates diet group (<20 g/day; -12.0 kg) compared to the caloric restricted diet (-6.5) [137]. Moreover, the low-carbohydrates diet group experienced a decrease in TG (-0,84 mmol/L *vs.* –0,31 mmol/L) and an increase in HDL-cholesterol levels (0,14 mmol/L *vs.* –0,04 mmol/L) compared to the low caloric diet. Recently, Foster et al have compared the efficacy of a carbohydrates restricted diet such as the Atkins diet versus a caloric restriction (1200-1500 kcal per day) in 63 obese subjects (mean body weight of 98 kg and BMI of 34 kg/m^2) [132]. The weight loss was more important in the "Atkins" group than the caloric restricted group after 6 months (7,6 *vs.* 2,7 kg respectively), but this weight loss was not different at 1 year (4,3 *vs.* 2,5 kg respectively) [132]. These two diets have a comparable impact after 12 months on blood pressure reduction and insulin response, and the "Atkins" diet was associated with a beneficial impact on triglycerides (a decrease of approximately 17 % from baseline after 1 year) and HDL-cholesterol (an increase of 11 % from baseline) [132]. The effects of a low-carbohydrates diet (<30 g per day, which was equivalent to a 250 ml orange juice in terms of grams of glucose) compared to the conventional low-fat diet (with a caloric deficit of 500 kcal/day) were also investigated in obese, type 2 diabetic and/or insulin-resistant subjects [134]. The intervention group had a greater loss of total body weight than the control group after 6 months of intervention (5,8 *vs.* 1,9 kg) [134]. A similar study was performed in 132 obese subjects (which included 83 % with MetS) randomly assigned to a low-carbohydrates diet or a caloric restriction of 500 kcal per day. These diet regimen did not induce a significant weight loss following 1-year of treatment [133]. Nevertheless, the lipid profile and glycemic control were improved in the low-carbohydrate group [133]. Some side effects were reported following the low-carbohydrate diet compared to the conventional low-fat diet such as constipation (68 % vs. 35 %), headaches (60 % vs. 40 %), muscular cramp (35 % vs. 7 %), diarrhea (23 % vs. 7 %) and general tiredness (25 % vs. 8 %) (137).

The Atkins Nutritional Approach

This weight loss regimen consists in a four step nutritional approach, including a 2-week introduction phase (Phase 1), an ongoing weight loss phase (Phase 2), a pre-maintenance phase (Phase 3) and, a lifetime maintenance phase (Phase 4) [130]. The diet "philosophy" of phase 1 is to induce a significant weight loss by reducing drastically carbohydrates consumption to stimulate fat metabolism via enhanced lipolysis while glycolysis will maintain adequate circulating blood glucose concentration [130]. The energetic intake from carbohydrates consists of a maximum of 20 g per day, primarily from salad and other non-starchy vegetables. This carbohydrate intake is clearly inferior to the dietary reference intakes from the NIH, the NAASO, the AHA and the NCEP-ATPIII, which correspond approximately to 180 g to 225 g per day for a daily energetic consumption of 1500 kcal [7;9;20;130]. Meat consumption (beef, fish, veal, eggs, poultry) is unlimited until satiety, cheese is limited to 90 g (which is equivalent to 3 slices of process cheese product), lettuce (salad, spinach or celery) to 500 ml/day, and vegetables low in carbohydrates (as broccoli and cauliflower) to 250 ml/day. Fruits, bread, pasta, rice, nuts and starchy vegetables such as potatoes must be avoided [130]. The utilisation of the GI of foods is also recommended in order to choose food with less influence on blood glucose level. During the second phase, the carbohydrate consumption is increased up to 25 g/day. Gradually, the net carbohydrate consumption is increased (5g-carbohydrates increment), until weight loss slows with less than 2.5 kg to 5 kg to be lost. The third phase begins when the participant approaches within 2.5

kg to 5 kg of the goal. Carbohydrates are increased weekly (5 g increment) as long as the subject continues to lose these last few kilos. Carbohydrates are increased until participants lose less than 0.5 kg per week [130]. The last phase (phase 4) recommends the steady daily consumption of carbohydrates, which was determined during the phase 3, in order to maintain weight loss.

Very-Low-Fat/Very-High-Carbohydrate Diet

A very low fat diet can be defined as one in which ≤15 % of total calories are derived from fat (equally distributed among saturated, monounsaturated and polyunsaturated fat). Approximately ≥70 % of total daily calories should be derived from carbohydrates and 15 % from protein. Even if very-low-fat diet may lead to important weight loss and improve lipid profile, they are not recommended for the general population since many studies have shown that weight loss is not sustained long term [138-141]. Moreover, in individuals with low HDL-cholesterol, high triglyceride and high insulin levels, it was reported that this kind of diet can amplify these abnormalities [141;142].

The Ornish Lifestyle Program

In contrast to the low-carbohydrates or the very-low-carbohydrates diets, the Ornish lifestyle program is rather a very low in fat and a very high carbohydrates diet [143]. Less than 10 % of total calories are from fat, 15 % from proteins and 75 % from complex carbohydrates, including a classification based on their starchy molecule, their chemical composition and their slower rate of carbohydrate absorption, as the GI of foods. A vegetarian diet, which includes eggs and low-fat dairy products, is suggested. It is also recommended to restrict cholesterol consumption to 100 mg daily and alcohol to less than 30 ml per day. Caffeine consumption is avoided and sodium is limited in the presence of hypertension, cardiovascular and renal disease. Physical activity, relaxation and meditation is strongly recommended. An observational study from Franklin et al has evaluated the adherence to the diet and nutrition component of a Ornish-type program on 10 subjects with CAD [144]. These patients followed a total vegetarian, very-low fat diet (10 % of total energy from fat) during 28 weeks. Weight loss ranged from 0.1 kg to 11.7 kg without beneficial impact on lipid values [144]. Moreover, only one subject had 100 % adherence to the dietary principles [144]. Aldana et al have compared the effects of the Ornish program to the traditional cardiac rehabilitation program or no rehabilitation at all on 84 subjects treated for CAD [145]. The nutritional programs and the follow-up were more extensive than the previous study, including approximately 5 hours of nutritional consultation per week. A significant reduction of anginal frequency, body weight, BMI, systolic blood pressure, total cholesterol, LDL cholesterol, glucose and dietary fat were observed on the Ornish group compared to the traditional rehabilitation program [145]. Table 5 presents a summary of the main differences in the macronutrient composition of most popular diets.

Table 5. Changes in the macronutrient composition of most popular diets

	Very-low-fat/very-high-carbohydrate diet	Low-carbohydrate/very-high-protein diets		Very-low-carbohydrate/very-high-protein/fat diets			
	The Ornish program (128)	The Montignac Method (107)		The Zone diet (111)	The South Beach Diet (109)	Atkins (111)	The Ornish program (128)
				Phase 1	Phase 2	Phase 3	
Total fat (% kcal)	**10**	32	29	62	43	39	68
Saturated fat	--	14	9	--	--	--	26
Carbohydrate (% kcal)	75	37	36	10	27	28	5
Protein (% kcal)	**15**	31	34	28	30	33	27
Alcohol (% kcal)	< 30 mL/day	--	1	A	A	A	--

Adapted from references 119, 122, 125, 130 and 143

Dietary Interventions Focusing on Lowering CHD Risk and Cholesterol Levels

Antioxidant Nutrients and CHD Risk

It is well establish that oxidative stress is an important feature in the development of atherosclerosis. Oxidative modifications significantly increase the atherogenicity of cholesterol enriched particle through LDL oxidation, and initiate a cascade of reactions that results in atherosclerosis [146;147]. Carotenoids are lipid-soluble antioxidants found in high concentration in many yellow and green fruits and vegetables. There are evidences suggesting that dietary antioxidants such as carotenoids may contribute to cardiovascular protection and lower CVD risk through inhibition of LDL oxidation and preservation of endothelial function [20;146;148]. There has been increasing interest in β-carotene, vitamin E (alpha-tocopherol) and vitamin C (ascorbic acid) supplementation regarding CVD benefits and cancer prevention [147;149-155]. Some data regarding consumption of antioxidant-rich foods, particularly vitamin E, support the hypothesis that carotenoids may exert their influence on the atherosclerotic process, preventing arterial plaque formation, particularly in individuals with the lowest intake. An inverse relation has been found between consumption of fruits, vegetables and whole grains and CVD [153-155]. However, results about the intake of carotenoids and vitamin E remain sparse [150;152-156]. There are even data suggesting that vitamin E supplementation has no apparent effect or may be detrimental regarding CVD and cancer (150;151;156). The Heart Outcomes Prevention Evaluation (HOPE) trial has reported a neutral effect of vitamin E, ingested either in food and in supplement, on CVD after 4.5 years of treatment in 9541 patients with high risk of CVD [151;156]. Recently, the HOPE-The Outgoing Outcomes (HOPE-TOO) trial performed on 3994 subjects has shown a 19 %

increase in heart failure and a 40 % increase in the risk of hospital admission for heart failure in patients receiving a long term supplementation with vitamin E (400 IU daily) [150]. Until now, there is insufficient evidence for recommendations regarding the use of antioxidants supplements [20]. A study of Moska et al has shown that a high dose combination of antioxidant nutrients (800 IU of vitamin E, 1000 mg of vitamin C and 24 mg of β-carotene) could inhibit the oxidative modification of LDL-cholesterol in patients with CVD [149]. Lycopene is a carotenoid without provitamin A activity and it is predominantly found in tomato-based foods, which is approximately 80 % of the lycopene intake in the American diet. Contrary to the other carotenoids, lycopene is more ubiquitous in fruits and vegetables. Lycopene has unique structural and chemical features, which permit the molecule to be resistant to cooking. Numerous studies have suggested a beneficial role of high plasma lycopene in the early stages of atherogenesis and CVD reduction which may have clinical and public health relevance in both men and women [148;157;158]. A decreased oxidative modification of LDL may be one the mechanism by which lycopene may reduce the risk of atherosclerotic progression and CVD risk [148;159].

Homocysteine and CHD Risk

In the last few years, there has been increasing interest in homocysteine, which has been considered as a predictor of CVD, particularly in patients with type 2 diabetes. Elevated levels of the amino acid are associated with increased risk of morbidity and mortality. Boushey et al have shown that approximately 10% of CAD risk may be attributed to hyperhomocysteinemia [160]. An increase of plasma homocysteine of 5 μmol/L could increase coronary risk 1.6-fold in men and 1.8-fold in women [160]. However, other studies have not confirmed the association between increased plasma homocysteine levels and CVD [161;162]. Moreover, the mechanism underlying the homocysteine related cardiovascular diseases remains unclear. Several dietary interventions, including various combinations of vitamins B6 and B12 with and without folic acid have reported a reduction of up to 50% in homocysteine levels [163]. Recently, a study performed on 609 subjects either with normal glucose metabolism, impaired glucose metabolism and type 2 diabetes has shown no association between homocysteine levels and cardiovascular autonomic function [164].

Soy Protein, Isoflavones and Cholesterol Levels

Soy protein consumption has been shown over the last 40 years to significantly decrease the risk of developing CHD [165] Recent research has examined dietary soy protein in the form of whole foods such as tofu, "soymilk," or as soy protein added to foods. Hence, recent studies have focused on the specific components of soy, such as the soy phytoestrogen isoflavones (genistein and daidzein). Soy protein has been associated with a lowering effect of 5 % to 6 % in LDL-cholesterol levels in response to protein substitution (animal for soy protein). A meta-analysis had shown that consuming a high vegetables protein diet in replacement of animal protein products can lower total cholesterol, LDL-cholesterol and triglycerides by 4-7 % without affecting HDL-cholesterol [166]. These effects were more important when baseline total cholesterol levels were ≥ 6.2 mmol/L [166]. Somehow, the effect on HDL-cholesterol level were inconsistent [167-171]. In moderately hypercholesterolemic men (total cholesterol concentration between 5.70 and 7.70 mmol/L), the consumption of 20 g to 50 g of soy protein per day induced a 3 % to 4.5 % decrease in non-HDL-cholesterol concentration [169]. The isoflavones fraction has been reported to have other lipid-independent positive effects, such as lowering blood pressure and increasing LDL oxidation resistance [165;172]. Moreover, phytoestrogen isoflavones have been largely associated with cholesterol reduction [168]. A study from Crouse and al has demonstrated that 62 mg of isoflavones (which correspond to approximately 30 g of whole soy) can decrease total cholesterol (9 %) and LDL-cholesterol (10 %) in hypercholesterolemic individuals compared to a casein diet [168]. The related effects in reducing total and LDL-cholesterol may be explained by the substitution of soy products, which are naturally low in saturated fat and cholesterol, for animal protein, which are high in these constituents. Since October 1999, the US Food and Drugs Administration (FDA) has approved a health claim about soy protein. Foods that contain more than 6.25 g of soy protein per serving (on the assumption of 4 servings per day or an intake of 25 g of soy protein daily) may help lower heart disease risk. Soy protein has been reviewed recently by the AHA [173].

Soluble Fibres and Cholesterol Levels

Soluble fibres such as oat bran, pectin and guar gum as well as viscous non-fermentable fibres such as psyllium are associated with decreased LDL-cholesterol and glucose levels (174-177). Current guidelines recommend to increase fibre intake to 25-30 g per day (current daily fibre intake in North America corresponds to approximately 10 to 15 g), with an emphasis on vegetables, cereals, whole grains and fruits [7;9;20]. The suggested mechanism by which soluble fibres lower cholesterol levels is the binding of bile acids in the intestinal lumen resulting in decreased absorption and increased fecal excretion of cholesterol [176]. The FDA has approved health claims for 2 dietary fibres, the β-glucan (0.75 g/serving) and psyllium (1.78 g/serving) in terms of reduction of CHD. Jenkins et al have assessed the efficacy of a high-fibre diet including 4 servings per day of foods containing β-glucan and psyllium that delivered 8 g of soluble fibres per day [174]. This high-fibre diet showed a significant 2.1 % decrease in total cholesterol, a 2.9 % increase in HDL-cholesterol and 1.4 % reduction in apo B/A-I ratio compared to the conventional low-fat/low-cholesterol diet [174]. The advantages of a high-fibre diet have also been assessed in type 2 diabetes. Besides their effect on serum lipid concentrations, soluble fibres such as psyllium have been shown to improve glycemic control (a 1.6 % decrease of HbA1c after 8 weeks of treatment with 5.1 g b.i.d. of psyllium husk fiber) [175].

Plant Sterols (Stanol/Sterol Esters) and Cholesterol Levels

Plant sterol and plant stanol esters have been documented to be effective in reducing total and LDL-cholesterol. The mechanism which explains the cholesterol lowering effects of plant sterols is by interference with the intestinal tract uptake of both dietary and biliary cholesterol in humans [178;179]. The NCEP-ATPIII recommends the addition of 2 g per day of plant sterols/stanols to the diet in patients at risk of CVD [7;180]. Plant sterols can be provided in small quantities in many fruits, vegetables, nuts, seeds, cereals, legumes, and other plant sources or incorporated into food products. The effectiveness of plant sterol/stanol added to foods such as margarine have reported a 15 % reduction in total and LDL-cholesterol [181-184]. The FDA has authorized use of labelling health claims about the positive role of plant sterol or plant stanol esters in reducing the risk of CHD regarding foods containing these substances. Moreover, intake of 2 to 3 g of plant sterols per day was shown to decrease total and LDL-cholesterol levels by 9 % to 20 % respectively, without altering HDL-cholesterol (182-185).

Considering the potential of functional ingredients recognized by the AHA and the NCEP-ATPIII, which now advocate the use of viscous fibers and plant sterols, soy protein and nuts, Jenkins et al have compared the effectiveness of these functional ingredients to the traditional first-generation statin treatment (lovastatin) on lipid profile [7;20;186]. The "portfolio" diet reduced LDL-cholesterol (30 %) and induced clinically significant reductions in the CHD risk. Interestingly, the dietary combination of these functional ingredients may not differ from the effect of first-generation statin regarding the achieved lipids target [186].

ω-3 Fatty Acids and Cholesterol Levels

Long-chain ω-3 fatty acids (omega-3) found in fish, EPA and DHA/fish oil and in omega-3 fatty acids supplements have been associated with beneficial effects either in animal model and in patients with and without CAD, particularly regarding mortality from CHD and sudden cardiac death [187-191]. Conflicting results have been reported in patients with an implantable cardioverter defibrillator assigned to receive omega-3 supplement, showing either protective or no effect on arrhythmic and cardiac death [192-194]. A recent study has shown that fish oil supplementation does not reduce the risk of ventricular tachycardia or ventricular fibrillation in this population, and may be proarrhythmic in some patients [192]. The potential mechanisms by which ω-3 fatty acids may reduce risk of CVD are not clear. Some hypothesis are: 1) reduced susceptibility to ventricular arrhythmia, 2) antithrombogenic effect, 3) nitric oxide-induced endothelial relaxation, 4) retarded atherosclerotic plaque growth, 5) hypotriglyceridemic effect and, 6) hypotensive effect [195]. Evidences suggest that two kinds of omega-3 fatty acids, eicosapentaenoic acid (EPA) and docosahexaenoic acid (DHA) supplementation from 0.5 to 1.8 g per day from fatty fish or supplements can significantly reduce subsequent cardiac and all-cause mortality [190]. The GISSI trial has reported a 20 % reduction in overall mortality and a 45 % reduction in sudden death after 3.5 years using a 850 mg dose of EPA and DHA ω-3 fatty acids supplementation (either with and without vitamin E) in subjects with preexisting CHD (187;189). The DART trial has reported a 29 % reduction in all-cause mortality over a 2-year period following the increase intake of fatty fish to 200-400 g per week in individuals with previous myocardial infarction [191]. Omega-3 fatty acids decrease TG levels by 25 % to 30 % with an associated increase of 1 % to 3 % in HDL-cholesterol and a 5 % to 10 % increase in LDL-cholesterol [196]. Current guidelines recommend at least 2 servings of fatty fish per week (such as mackerel, lake trout, herring, sardines, albacore tuna and salmon), in conjunction with the inclusion of vegetable oils and food sources high in α-linolenic acids (canola, soybean oils, flaxseed, walnuts) for most individuals [20;190]. In patients with documented CVD, EPA and DHA supplements could be considered in addition with the consumption of 1 g daily of EPA+DHA from varied fatty fish. In patients with high levels of TG, 2 to 4 g of EPA+DHA daily are recommended, ideally from supplements under medical supervision [190]).

CONCLUSION

Lifestyle and dietary modifications are important strategies in the management of obesity, hypertension, CVD and MetS. Achieving normal lipoprotein profile, body weight and BP is primordial in the prevention and treatment of CVD. Conventional dietary guidelines provide nutritional recommendations; together with other healthy practices such as regular physical exercise and smoking cessation, to reduce health complications. Since some popular diets such as the very-low-fat diet or the high protein diet have challenged the effectiveness of conventional low-fat diet, further studies will be needed to establish the ideal macronutrient intake to achieve long-term weight reduction and health benefit. In conjunction with a suitable energy intake for maintaining a normal body weight, optimal carbohydrate, protein and fat dietary ratio should be determined to improve insulin sensitivity and lipids profile. These different diets seem to have variable short-term positive effects on weight reduction and lipids profile. Recently, Dansinger et al have assessed the adherence rates and the effectiveness of four popular diets (Atkins, Zone, Weight Watchers, and Ornish) for weight loss and cardiac risk factor reduction on 160 individuals [139]. Even if there was a significant reduction of total daily calories intake and body weight in all groups, each popular diet modestly reduced body weight and cardiac risk factors at 1 year. More importantly, this study demonstrated that long-term overall dietary adherence and maintenance were low using extreme macronutrient intake, since 42 % of the participants dropped out during this 1-year study [139]. Actually, these types of diets do not seem to have advantages over the conventional diets at one year, and the observance to these nutritional modifications is often difficult. The ideal treatment for long-term abdominal obesity, hypertension, CVD and MetS should be individualized, intensive and under the supervision of qualified health care professionals. There is no bad diet; the only good one is the one that will permit to achieve long-term weight balance and can contribute to reduce hypertension, CVD and MetS without nutrient deficit as well as all other risks.

REFERENCES

[1] Belanger-Ducharme F, Tremblay A. Prevalence of obesity in Canada. *Obes Rev* 2005; 6(3):183-186.

[2] Mokdad AH, Bowman BA, Ford ES, Vinicor F, Marks JS, Koplan JP. The continuing epidemics of obesity and diabetes in the United States. *JAMA* 2001; 286(10):1195-1200.

[3] Baskin ML, Ard J, Franklin F, Allison DB. Prevalence of obesity in the United States. *Obes Rev* 2005; 6(1):5-7.

[4] Pérusse L, Bouchard C. Gene-diet interactions in obesity. *Am J Clin Nutr* 2000; 72(5 Suppl):1285S-1290S.

[5] Yusuf S, Hawken S, Ounpuu S, Bautista L, Franzosi MG, Commerford P et al. Obesity and the risk of myocardial infarction in 27,000 participants from 52 countries: a case-control study. *Lancet* 2005; 366(9497):1640-1649.

[6] Grundy SM, Cleeman JI, Daniels SR, Donato KA, Eckel RH, Franklin BA et al. Diagnosis and management of the metabolic syndrome: an American Heart Association/National Heart, Lung, and Blood Institute Scientific Statement. *Circulation* 2005; 112(17):2735-2752.

[7] The National Cholesterol Education Program - Adult Treatment Panel III. Executive Summary of The Third Report of The National Cholesterol Education Program (NCEP) Expert Panel on Detection, Evaluation, And Treatment of High Blood Cholesterol In Adults (Adult Treatment Panel III). *JAMA* 2001; 285(19):2486-2497.

[8] Eckel RH, Krauss RM. American Heart Association call to action: obesity as a major risk factor for coronary heart disease. AHA Nutrition Committee. *Circulation* 1998; 97(21):2099-2100.

[9] National Institutes of Health. The Pratical Guide Indentification, Evaluation and Treatment of Overweight and Obesity in Adults. *National Health, lung and blood institute North American Association for the Study of Obesity* 2002;1-80.

[10] Wing RR, Koeske R, Epstein LH, Nowalk MP, Gooding W, Becker D. Long-term effects of modest weight loss in type II diabetic patients. *Arch Intern Med* 1987; 147(10):1749-1753.

[11] Mertens IL, Van Gaal LF. Overweight, obesity, and blood pressure: the effects of modest weight reduction. *Obes Res* 2000; 8(3):270-278.

[12] Blackburn G. Effect of degree of weight loss on health benefits. *Obes Res* 1995; 3 Suppl 2:211s-216s.

[13] Alberti KG, Zimmet PZ. Definition, diagnosis and classification of diabetes mellitus and its complications. Part 1: diagnosis and classification of diabetes mellitus provisional report of a WHO consultation. *Diabet Med* 1998; 15(7):539-553.

[14] Isomaa B, Almgren P, Tuomi T, Forsen B, Lahti K, Nissen M et al. Cardiovascular morbidity and mortality associated with the metabolic syndrome. *Diabetes Care* 2001; 24(4):683-689.

[15] Eckel RH, Barouch WW, Ershow AG. Report of the National Heart, Lung, and Blood Institute-National Institute of Diabetes and Digestive and Kidney Diseases Working Group on the pathophysiology of obesity-associated cardiovascular disease. *Circulation* 2002; 105(24):2923-2928.

[16] Report of a WHO consultation. Definition of metabolic syndrome in definition, diagnosis, and classification of diabetes mellitus and its complications. Part I: Diagnosis and classification of diabetes mellitus. Alwan A, King H, 1996. World Health Organisation, pp 1-59.

[17] International Diabetes Federation. The IDF Consensus Worldwide Definition of the Metabolic Syndrome. International Diabetes Federation, editor. 2005. Brussels, Belgium, International Diabetes Federation, pp 1-7.

[18] Ford ES, Giles WH, Dietz WH. Prevalence of the metabolic syndrome among US adults: findings from the third National Health and Nutrition Examination Survey. *JAMA* 2002; 287(3):356-359.

[19] Wilson PW, Grundy SM. The metabolic syndrome: practical guide to origins and treatment: Part I. *Circulation* 2003; 108(12):1422-1424.

[20] Krauss RM, Eckel RH, Howard B, Appel LJ, Daniels SR, Deckelbaum RJ et al. AHA Dietary Guidelines: revision 2000: A statement for healthcare professionals from the Nutrition Committee of the American Heart Association. *Circulation* 2000; 102(18):2284-2299.

[21] Després JP. Abdominal obesity and the risk of coronary artery disease. *Can J Cardiol* 1992; 8(6):561-562.

[22] Pouliot MC, Després JP, Nadeau A, Moorjani S, Prud'homme D, Lupien PJ et al. Visceral obesity in men. Associations with glucose tolerance, plasma insulin, and lipoprotein levels. *Diabetes* 1992; 41(7):826-834.

[23] Després JP, Moorjani S, Lupien PJ, Tremblay A, Nadeau A, Bouchard C. Regional distribution of body fat, plasma lipoproteins, and cardiovascular disease. *Arteriosclerosis* 1990; 10(4):497-511.

[24] Poirier P, Després JP. Waist circumference, visceral obesity, and cardiovascular risk. *J Cardiopulm Rehabil* 2003; 23(3):161-169.

[25] Poirier P, Eckel RH. Obesity and cardiovascular disease. *Curr Atheroscler Rep* 2002; 4(6):448-453.

[26] Dagenais GR, Yi Q, Mann JF, Bosch J, Pogue J, Yusuf S. Prognostic impact of body weight and abdominal obesity in women and men with cardiovascular disease. *Am Heart J* 2005; 149(1):54-60.

[27] World Health Organization. Obesity: Preventing and Managing the Global Epidemic. WHO technical report series no. 894. 2000. Geneva, World Health Organisation.

[28] Health Canada. Canadian guidelines for body weight classification in adults. 2003. Ottawa.

[29] Lemieux I, Pascot A, Couillard C, Lamarche B, Tchernof A, Almeras N et al. Hypertriglyceridemic waist: A marker of the atherogenic metabolic triad (hyperinsulinemia; hyperapolipoprotein B; small, dense LDL) in men? *Circulation* 2000; 102(2):179-184.

[30] Janssen I, Katzmarzyk PT, Ross R. Body mass index, waist circumference, and health risk: evidence in support of current National Institutes of Health guidelines. *Arch Intern Med* 2002; 162(18):2074-2079.

[31] Burt VL, Whelton P, Roccella EJ, Brown C, Cutler JA, Higgins M et al. Prevalence of hypertension in the US adult population. Results from the Third National Health and Nutrition Examination Survey, 1988-1991. *Hypertension* 1995; 25(3):305-313.

[32] Appel LJ, Moore TJ, Obarzanek E, Vollmer WM, Svetkey LP, Sacks FM et al. A clinical trial of the effects of dietary patterns on blood pressure. DASH Collaborative Research Group. *N Engl J Med* 1997; 336(16):1117-1124.

[33] Khan NA, McAlister FA, Lewanczuk RZ, Touyz RM, Padwal R, Rabkin SW et al. The 2005 Canadian Hypertension Education Program recommendations for the management of hypertension: part II - therapy. *Can J Cardiol* 2005; 21(8):657-672.

[34] Yusuf S, Hawken S, Ounpuu S, Dans T, Avezum A, Lanas F et al. Effect of potentially modifiable risk factors associated with myocardial infarction in 52 countries (the INTERHEART study): case-control study. *Lancet* 2004; 364:937-952.

[35] Poirier P, Lemieux I, Mauriège P, Dewailly E, Blanchet C, Bergeron J et al. Impact of Waist Circumference on the Relationship Between Blood Pressure and Insulin. The Quebec Health Survey. *Hypertension* 2005.

[36] Macdonald SM, Reeder BA, Chen Y, Despres JP. Obesity in Canada: a descriptive analysis. Canadian Heart Health Surveys Research Group. *CMAJ* 1997; 157 Suppl 1:S3-S9.

[37] Johnson D, Prud'homme D, Després JP, Nadeau A, Tremblay A, Bouchard C. Relation of abdominal obesity to hyperinsulinemia and high blood pressure in men. *Int J Obes Relat Metab Disord* 1992; 16(11):881-890.

[38] Riccardi G, Giacco R, Rivellese AA. Dietary fat, insulin sensitivity and the metabolic syndrome. *Clin Nutr* 2004; 23(4):447-456.

[39] Klein S, Burke LE, Bray GA, Blair S, Allison DB, Pi-Sunyer X et al. Clinical implications of obesity with specific focus on cardiovascular disease: a statement for professionals from the American Heart Association Council on Nutrition, Physical Activity, and Metabolism: endorsed by the American College of Cardiology Foundation. *Circulation* 2004; 110(18):2952-2967.

[40] Riccardi G, Rivellese AA. Dietary treatment of the metabolic syndrome--the optimal diet. *Br J Nutr* 2000; 83 Suppl 1:S143-S148.

[41] US Department of Health and Human Services. Physical Activity and Health: A Report of the Surgeon General Executive Summary. Center for Disease Control and Prevention, 1996, pp 1-18.

[42] Pate RR, Pratt M, Blair SN, Haskell WL, Macera CA, Bouchard C et al. Physical activity and public health. A recommendation from the Centers for Disease Control and Prevention and the American College of Sports Medicine. *JAMA* 1995; 273(5):402-407.

[43] Tremblay A, Lavallée N, Almeras N, Allard L, Després JP, Bouchard C. Nutritional determinants of the increase in energy intake associated with a high-fat diet. *Am J Clin Nutr* 1991; 53(5):1134-1137.

[44] Vollmer WM, Sacks FM, Ard J, Appel LJ, Bray GA, Simons-Morton DG et al. Effects of diet and sodium intake on blood pressure: subgroup analysis of the DASH-sodium trial. *Ann Intern Med* 2001; 135(12):1019-1028.

[45] Sacks FM, Svetkey LP, Vollmer WM, Appel LJ, Bray GA, Harsha D et al. Effects on blood pressure of reduced dietary sodium and the Dietary Approaches to Stop Hypertension (DASH) diet. DASH-Sodium Collaborative Research Group. *N Engl J Med* 2001; 344(1):3-10.

[46] Poston WS, Haddock CK, Dill PL, Thayer B, Foreyt JP. Lifestyle treatments in randomized clinical trials of pharmacotherapies for obesity. *Obes Res* 2001; 9(9):552-563.

[47] Wadden TA. Treatment of obesity by moderate and severe caloric restriction. Results of clinical research trials. *Ann Intern Med* 1993; 119(7 Pt 2):688-693.

[48] Wadden TA, Foster GD, Letizia KA. One-year behavioral treatment of obesity: comparison of moderate and severe caloric restriction and the effects of weight maintenance therapy. *J Consult Clin Psychol* 1994; 62(1):165-171.

[49] Isner JM, Sours HE, Paris AL, Ferrans VJ, Roberts WC. Sudden, unexpected death in avid dieters using the liquid-protein-modified-fast diet. Observations in 17 patients and the role of the prolonged QT interval. *Circulation* 1979; 60(6):1401-1412.

[50] Frank S, Colliver JA, Frank A. Low-energy diets and prolonged QT intervals. *JAMA* 1987; 257(12):1601-1602.

[51] Doherty JU, Wadden TA, Zuk L, Letizia KA, Foster GD, Day SC. Long-term evaluation of cardiac function in obese patients treated with a very-low-calorie diet: a controlled clinical study of patients without underlying cardiac disease. *Am J Clin Nutr* 1991; 53(4):854-858.

[52] Moyer C.L., Holly R.H., Amsterdam E.A., Atkinson R.L. Effects of cardiac stress during a very-low-calorie diet and exercise program in obese women. *American Journal of Clinical Nutrition* 1989; 50:1324-1327.

[53] Wang Y, Wang QJ. The prevalence of prehypertension and hypertension among US adults according to the new joint national committee guidelines: new challenges of the old problem. *Arch Intern Med* 2004; 164(19):2126-2134.

[54] Lauber RP, Sheard NF. The American Heart Association Dietary Guidelines for 2000: a summary report. *Nutr Rev* 2001; 59(9):298-306.

[55] Svetkey LP, Sacks FM, Obarzanek E, Vollmer WM, Appel LJ, Lin PH et al. The DASH Diet, Sodium Intake and Blood Pressure Trial (DASH-sodium): rationale and design. DASH-Sodium Collaborative Research Group. *J Am Diet Assoc* 1999; 99(8 Suppl):S96-104.

[56] Zemel MB. Dietary pattern and hypertension: the DASH study. Dietary Approaches to Stop Hypertension. *Nutr Rev* 1997; 55(8):303-305.

[57] Chobanian AV, Bakris GL, Black HR, Cushman WC, Green LA, Izzo JL, Jr. et al. The Seventh Report of the Joint National Committee on Prevention, Detection, Evaluation, and Treatment of High Blood Pressure: the JNC 7 report. *JAMA* 2003; 289(19):2560-2572.

[58] European Society of Hypertension-European Society of Cardiology. 2003 European Society of Hypertension-European Society of Cardiology guidelines for the management of arterial hypertension. *J Hypertens* 2003; 21(6):1011-1053.

[59] De Lorgeril M, Salen P, Martin JL, Monjaud I, Delaye J, Mamelle N. Mediterranean diet, traditional risk factors, and the rate of cardiovascular complications after myocardial infarction: final report of the Lyon Diet Heart Study. *Circulation* 1999; 99(6):779-785.

[60] Appel LJ, Sacks FM, Carey VJ, Obarzanek E, Swain JF, Miller ER, III et al. Effects of Protein, Monounsaturated Fat, and Carbohydrate Intake on Blood Pressure and Serum Lipids: Results of the OmniHeart Randomized Trial. *JAMA* 2005; 294(19):2455-2464.

[61] Kelley DE, Goodpaster BH. Effects of exercise on glucose homeostasis in Type 2 diabetes mellitus. *Med Sci Sports Exerc* 2001; 33(6 Suppl):S495-S501.

[62] Moore LL, Visioni AJ, Wilson PW, D'Agostino RB, Finkle WD, Ellison RC. Can sustained weight loss in overweight individuals reduce the risk of diabetes mellitus? *Epidemiology* 2000; 11(3):269-273.

[63] Hollenbeck CB. Dietary fructose effects on lipoprotein metabolism and risk for coronary artery disease. *Am J Clin Nutr* 1993; 58(5 Suppl):800S-809S.

[64] Marshall JA, Hoag S, Shetterly S, Hamman RF. Dietary fat predicts conversion from impaired glucose tolerance to NIDDM. The San Luis Valley Diabetes Study. *Diabetes Care* 1994; 17(1):50-56.

[65] Matsuda M, Defronzo RA, Glass L, Consoli A, Giordano M, Bressler P et al. Glucagon dose-response curve for hepatic glucose production and glucose disposal in type 2 diabetic patients and normal individuals. *Metabolism* 2002; 51(9):1111-1119.

[66] Esposito K, Marfella R, Ciotola M, Di Palo C, Giugliano F, Giugliano G et al. Effect of a mediterranean-style diet on endothelial dysfunction and markers of vascular inflammation in the metabolic syndrome: a randomized trial. *JAMA* 2004; 292(12):1440-1446.

[67] Keys A, Menotti A, Karvonen MJ, Aravanis C, Blackburn H, Buzina R et al. The diet and 15-year death rate in the seven countries study. *Am J Epidemiol* 1986; 124(6):903-915.

[68] De Lorgeril M, Renaud S, Mamelle N, Salen P, Martin JL, Monjaud I et al. Mediterranean alpha-linolenic acid-rich diet in secondary prevention of coronary heart disease. *Lancet* 1994; 343(8911):1454-1459.

[69] Willett WC, Sacks F, Trichopoulou A, Drescher G, Ferro-Luzzi A, Helsing E et al. Mediterranean diet pyramid: a cultural model for healthy eating. *Am J Clin Nutr* 1995; 61(6 Suppl):1402S-1406S.

[70] Kris-Etherton P, Eckel RH, Howard BV, St Jeor S, Bazzarre TL. AHA Science Advisory: Lyon Diet Heart Study. Benefits of a Mediterranean-style, National Cholesterol Education Program/American Heart Association Step I Dietary Pattern on Cardiovascular Disease. *Circulation* 2001; 103(13):1823-1825.

[71] Goulet J, Lamarche B, Charest A, Nadeau G, Lapointe A, Desroches S et al. Effect of a nutritional intervention promoting the Mediterranean food pattern on electrophoretic characteristics of low-density lipoprotein particles in healthy women from the Quebec City metropolitan area. *Br J Nutr* 2004; 92(2):285-293.

[72] Lapointe A, Goulet J, Couillard C, Lamarche B, Lemieux S. A nutritional intervention promoting the Mediterranean food pattern is associated with a decrease in circulating oxidized LDL particles in healthy women from the Quebec City metropolitan area. *J Nutr* 2005; 135(3):410-415.

[73] Goulet J, Lamarche B, Nadeau G, Lemieux S. Effect of a nutritional intervention promoting the Mediterranean food pattern on plasma lipids, lipoproteins and body weight in healthy French-Canadian women. *Atherosclerosis* 2003; 170(1):115-124.

[74] Heshka S, Greenway F, Anderson JW, Atkinson RL, Hill JO, Phinney SD et al. Self-help weight loss versus a structured commercial program after 26 weeks: a randomized controlled study. *Am J Med* 2000; 109(4):282-287.

[75] Djuric Z, DiLaura NM, Jenkins I, Darga L, Jen CK, Mood D et al. Combining weight-loss counseling with the weight watchers plan for obese breast cancer survivors. *Obes Res* 2002; 10(7):657-665.

[76] Rippe JM, Price JM, Hess SA, Kline G, DeMers KA, Damitz S et al. Improved psychological well-being, quality of life, and health practices in moderately overweight women participating in a 12-week structured weight loss program. *Obes Res* 1998; 6(3):208-218.

[77] Lowe MR, Miller-Kovach K, Phelan S. Weight-loss maintenance in overweight individuals one to five years following successful completion of a commercial weight loss program. *Int J Obes Relat Metab Disord* 2001; 25(3):325-331.

[78] Frost G, Keogh B, Smith D, Akinsanya K, Leeds A. The effect of low-glycemic carbohydrate on insulin and glucose response in vivo and in vitro in patients with coronary heart disease. *Metabolism* 1996; 45(6):669-672.
[79] Schulze MB, Hu FB. Dietary approaches to prevent the metabolic syndrome: quality versus quantity of carbohydrates. *Diabetes Care* 2004; 27(2):613-614.
[80] FAO, WHO. Carbohydrates in humain nutrition. *FAO Food and nutrition paper* 1998; 66 (Rome):FAO.
[81] Nantel G. Glycemic carbohydrate: an international perspective. *Nutr Rev* 2003; 61(5 Pt 2):S34-S39.
[82] Canadian Diabetes Association. Clinical Practice Guidelines for the Prevention and Management of Diabetes in Canada. Canadian Journal of Diabetes 27[Supplement 2], 1-163. 2003.
[83] Franz MJ, Bantle JP, Beebe CA, Brunzell JD, Chiasson JL, Garg A et al. Nutrition principles and recommendations in diabetes. *Diabetes Care* 2004; 27 Suppl 1:S36-S46.
[84] Jenkins DJ, Wolever TM, Taylor RH, Barker H, Fielden H, Baldwin JM et al. Glycemic index of foods: a physiological basis for carbohydrate exchange. *Am J Clin Nutr* 1981; 34(3):362-366.
[85] Wolever TM, Jenkins DJ, Jenkins AL, Josse RG. The glycemic index: methodology and clinical implications. *Am J Clin Nutr* 1991; 54(5):846-854.
[86] Wolever TM, Vorster HH, Bjorck I, Brand-Miller J, Brighenti F, Mann JI et al. Determination of the glycaemic index of foods: interlaboratory study. *Eur J Clin Nutr* 2003; 57(3):475-482.
[87] Brand JC, Nicholson PL, Thorburn AW, Truswell AS. Food processing and the glycemic index. *Am J Clin Nutr* 1985; 42(6):1192-1196.
[88] Augustin LS, Franceschi S, Jenkins DJ, Kendall CW, La Vecchia C. Glycemic index in chronic disease: a review. *Eur J Clin Nutr* 2002; 56(11):1049-1071.
[89] Pi-Sunyer FX. Glycemic index and disease. *Am J Clin Nutr* 2002; 76(1):290S-298S.
[90] Jenkins AL, Jenkins DJ, Zdravkovic U, Wursch P, Vuksan V. Depression of the glycemic index by high levels of beta-glucan fiber in two functional foods tested in type 2 diabetes. *Eur J Clin Nutr* 2002; 56(7):622-628.
[91] Rizkalla SW, Bellisle F, Slama G. Health benefits of low glycaemic index foods, such as pulses, in diabetic patients and healthy individuals. *Br J Nutr* 2002; 88 Suppl 3:S255-S262.
[92] Kelley DE. Sugars and starch in the nutritional management of diabetes mellitus. *Am J Clin Nutr* 2003; 78(4):858S-864S.
[93] Heilbronn LK, Noakes M, Clifton PM. The effect of high- and low-glycemic index energy restricted diets on plasma lipid and glucose profiles in type 2 diabetic subjects with varying glycemic control. *J Am Coll Nutr* 2002; 21(2):120-127.
[94] Brand-Miller J, Hayne S, Petocz P, Colagiuri S. Low-glycemic index diets in the management of diabetes: a meta-analysis of randomized controlled trials. *Diabetes Care* 2003; 26(8):2261-2267.
[95] Willett W, Manson J, Liu S. Glycemic index, glycemic load, and risk of type 2 diabetes. *Am J Clin Nutr* 2002; 76(1):274S-280S.
[96] Ford ES, Liu S. Glycemic index and serum high-density lipoprotein cholesterol concentration among us adults. *Arch Intern Med* 2001; 161(4):572-576.

[97] Jenkins DJ, Wolever TM, Kalmusky J, Giudici S, Giordano C, Wong GS et al. Low glycemic index carbohydrate foods in the management of hyperlipidemia. *Am J Clin Nutr* 1985; 42(4):604-617.

[98] Jenkins DJ, Jenkins AL. The glycemic index, fiber, and the dietary treatment of hypertriglyceridemia and diabetes. *J Am Coll Nutr* 1987; 6(1):11-17.

[99] Ball SD, Keller KR, Moyer-Mileur LJ, Ding YW, Donaldson D, Jackson WD. Prolongation of satiety after low versus moderately high glycemic index meals in obese adolescents. *Pediatrics* 2003; 111(3):488-494.

[100] Roberts SB. Glycemic index and satiety. *Nutr Clin Care* 2003; 6(1):20-26.

[101] Brand-Miller JC, Holt SH, Pawlak DB, McMillan J. Glycemic index and obesity. *Am J Clin Nutr* 2002; 76(1):281S-285S.

[102] Ludwig DS, Majzoub JA, Al Zahrani A, Dallal GE, Blanco I, Roberts SB. High glycemic index foods, overeating, and obesity. Pediatrics 103[3], E26. 1999.

[103] Anderson GH, Woodend D. Effect of glycemic carbohydrates on short-term satiety and food intake. *Nutr Rev* 2003; 61(5 Pt 2):S17-S26.

[104] Warren JM, Henry CJ, Simonite V. Low glycemic index breakfasts and reduced food intake in preadolescent children. *Pediatrics* 2003; 112(5):e414-e419.

[105] Liu S, Willett WC, Stampfer MJ, Hu FB, Franz M, Sampson L et al. A prospective study of dietary glycemic load, carbohydrate intake, and risk of coronary heart disease in US women. *Am J Clin Nutr* 2000; 71(6):1455-1461.

[106] Salmeron J, Ascherio A, Rimm EB, Colditz GA, Spiegelman D, Jenkins DJ et al. Dietary fiber, glycemic load, and risk of NIDDM in men. *Diabetes Care* 1997; 20(4):545-550.

[107] Salmeron J, Manson JE, Stampfer MJ, Colditz GA, Wing AL, Willett WC. Dietary fiber, glycemic load, and risk of non-insulin-dependent diabetes mellitus in women. *JAMA* 1997; 277(6):472-477.

[108] Ludwig DS. Dietary glycemic index and the regulation of body weight. *Lipids* 2003; 38(2):117-121.

[109] Schulze MB, Hu FB. Dietary approaches to prevent the metabolic syndrome: quality versus quantity of carbohydrates. *Diabetes Care* 2004; 27(2):613-614.

[110] Kopp W. High-insulinogenic nutrition--an etiologic factor for obesity and the metabolic syndrome? *Metabolism* 2003; 52(7):840-844.

[111] Arner P. Control of lipolysis and its relevance to development of obesity in man. *Diabetes Metab Rev* 1988; 4(5):507-515.

[112] Saris WH. Sugars, energy metabolism, and body weight control. *Am J Clin Nutr* 2003; 78(4):850S-857S.

[113] Ball SD, Keller KR, Moyer-Mileur LJ, Ding YW, Donaldson D, Jackson WD. Prolongation of satiety after low versus moderately high glycemic index meals in obese adolescents. *Pediatrics* 2003; 111(3):488-494.

[114] Foster-Powell K, Holt SH, Brand-Miller JC. International table of glycemic index and glycemic load values: 2002. *Am J Clin Nutr* 2002; 76(1):5-56.

[115] Augustin LS, Franceschi S, Jenkins DJ, Kendall CW, La Vecchia C. Glycemic index in chronic disease: a review. *Eur J Clin Nutr* 2002; 56(11):1049-1071.

[116] Ludwig DS, Eckel RH. The glycemic index at 20 y. *Am J Clin Nutr* 2002; 76(1):264S-265S.

[117] Pawlak DB, Ebbeling CB, Ludwig DS. Spirited critique of glycaemic index (GI) and its role in the treatment of obesity. *Obes Rev* 2003; 4(1):73-74.

[118] Raben A. Should obese patients be counselled to follow a low-glycaemic index diet? No. *Obes Rev* 2002; 3(4):245-256.

[119] Montignac M. Je mange, je maigris et je reste mince! Flammarion (eds). *La méthode Montignac* 1999. Paris: J'ai Lu Publisher, pp9-318.

[120] Dumesnil JG, Montignac M. *Bon poids bon coeur avec la méthode Montignac* 2002. Flammarion (eds). Québec,.pp 15-269.

[121] Dumesnil JG, Turgeon J, Tremblay A, Poirier P, Gilbert M, Gagnon L et al. Effect of a low-glycaemic index--low-fat--high protein diet on the atherogenic metabolic risk profile of abdominally obese men. *Br J Nutr* 2001; 86(5):557-568.

[122] Agastston A. The delicious, doctor-designed, foolproof plan for fast and healthy weight lost. *The South Beach Diet* 2003. St-Martin's Griffin (eds); New York: St-Martin Press, pp 3-297.

[123] Aude YW, Agatston AS, Lopez-Jimenez F, Lieberman EH, Marie A, Hansen M et al. The national cholesterol education program diet vs a diet lower in carbohydrates and higher in protein and monounsaturated fat: a randomized trial. *Arch Intern Med* 2004; 164(19):2141-2146.

[124] St Jeor ST, Howard BV, Prewitt TE, Bovee V, Bazzarre T, Eckel RH. Dietary protein and weight reduction: a statement for healthcare professionals from the Nutrition Committee of the Council on Nutrition, Physical Activity, and Metabolism of the American Heart Association. *Circulation* 2001; 104(15):1869-1874.

[125] Sears B, Lawren B. Zone:Revolutionary life plan. *Enter the Zone* 1995. Canada: Harper Collins Publisher, pp 1-288.

[126] Miyashita Y, Koide N, Ohtsuka M, Ozaki H, Itoh Y, Oyama T et al. Beneficial effect of low carbohydrate in low calorie diets on visceral fat reduction in type 2 diabetic patients with obesity. *Diabetes Res Clin Pract* 2004; 65(3):235-241.

[127] Gulliford MC, Bicknell EJ, Scarpello JH. Differential effect of protein and fat ingestion on blood glucose responses to high- and low-glycemic-index carbohydrates in noninsulin-dependent diabetic subjects. *Am J Clin Nutr* 1989; 50(4):773-777.

[128] Tremblay A. Nutritional determinants of the insulin resistance syndrome. *Int J Obes Relat Metab Disord* 1995; 19 Suppl 1:S60-S68.

[129] Gannon MC, Nuttall FQ, Saeed A, Jordan K, Hoover H. An increase in dietary protein improves the blood glucose response in persons with type 2 diabetes. *Am J Clin Nutr* 2003; 78(4):734-741.

[130] Atkins RC. Dr Atkins' new diet revolution. *The Atkins Diet* 1998. New York: Harper Collins Publisher, pp3-560.

[131] A critique of low-carbohydrate ketogenic weight reduction regimens. A review of Dr. Atkins' diet revolution. *JAMA* 1973; 224(10):1415-1419.

[132] Foster GD, Wyatt HR, Hill JO, McGuckin BG, Brill C, Mohammed BS et al. A randomized trial of a low-carbohydrate diet for obesity. *N Engl J Med* 2003; 348(21):2082-2090.

[133] Stern L, Iqbal N, Seshadri P, Chicano KL, Daily DA, McGrory J et al. The effects of low-carbohydrate versus conventional weight loss diets in severely obese adults: one-year follow-up of a randomized trial. *Ann Intern Med* 2004; 140(10):778-785.

[134] Samaha FF, Iqbal N, Seshadri P, Chicano KL, Daily DA, McGrory J et al. A low-carbohydrate as compared with a low-fat diet in severe obesity. *N Engl J Med* 2003; 348(21):2074-2081.

[135] Westman EC, Yancy WS, Edman JS, Tomlin KF, Perkins CE. Effect of 6-month adherence to a very low carbohydrate diet program. *Am J Med* 2002; 113(1):30-36.

[136] Lara-Castro C, Garvey WT. Diet, insulin resistance, and obesity: zoning in on data for Atkins dieters living in South Beach. *J Clin Endocrinol Metab* 2004; 89(9):4197-4205.

[137] Yancy WS, Jr., Olsen MK, Guyton JR, Bakst RP, Westman EC. A low-carbohydrate, ketogenic diet versus a low-fat diet to treat obesity and hyperlipidemia: a randomized, controlled trial. *Ann Intern Med* 2004; 140(10):769-777.

[138] Lichtenstein AH, Van Horn L. Very low fat diets. *Circulation* 1998; 98(9):935-939.

[139] Dansinger ML, Gleason JA, Griffith JL, Selker HP, Schaefer EJ. Comparison of the Atkins, Ornish, Weight Watchers, and Zone diets for weight loss and heart disease risk reduction: a randomized trial. *JAMA* 2005; 293(1):43-53.

[140] Sheppard L, Kristal AR, Kushi LH. Weight loss in women participating in a randomized trial of low-fat diets. *Am J Clin Nutr* 1991; 54(5):821-828.

[141] Kasim-Karakas SE, Almario RU, Mueller WM, Peerson J. Changes in plasma lipoproteins during low-fat, high-carbohydrate diets: effects of energy intake. *Am J Clin Nutr* 2000; 71(6):1439-1447.

[142] Chen YD, Coulston AM, Zhou MY, Hollenbeck CB, Reaven GM. Why do low-fat high-carbohydrate diets accentuate postprandial lipemia in patients with NIDDM? *Diabetes Care* 1995; 18(1):10-16.

[143] Ornish D. *Dr Dean Ornish's Program for Reversion Heart Disease* 1992. New York: Ivy Publisher, pp 3-672.

[144] Franklin TL, Kolasa KM, Griffin K, Mayo C, Badenhop DT. Adherence to very-low-fat diet by a group of cardiac rehabilitation patients in the rural southeastern United States. *Arch Fam Med* 1995; 4(6):551-554.

[145] Aldana SG, Whitmer WR, Greenlaw R, Avins AL, Salberg A, Barnhurst M et al. Cardiovascular risk reductions associated with aggressive lifestyle modification and cardiac rehabilitation. *Heart Lung* 2003; 32(6):374-382.

[146] Gaziano JM, Manson JE, Branch LG, Colditz GA, Willett WC, Buring JE. A prospective study of consumption of carotenoids in fruits and vegetables and decreased cardiovascular mortality in the elderly. *Ann Epidemiol* 1995; 5(4):255-260.

[147] Manson JE, Gaziano JM, Spelsberg A, Ridker PM, Cook NR, Buring JE et al. A secondary prevention trial of antioxidant vitamins and cardiovascular disease in women. Rationale, design, and methods. The WACS Research Group. *Ann Epidemiol* 1995; 5(4):261-269.

[148] Rissanen T, Voutilainen S, Nyyssonen K, Salonen JT. Lycopene, atherosclerosis, and coronary heart disease. *Exp Biol Med (Maywood)* 2002; 227(10):900-907.

[149] Mosca L, Rubenfire M, Mandel C, Rock C, Tarshis T, Tsai A et al. Antioxidant nutrient supplementation reduces the susceptibility of low density lipoprotein to oxidation in patients with coronary artery disease. *J Am Coll Cardiol* 1997; 30(2):392-399.

[150] Lonn E, Bosch J, Yusuf S, Sheridan P, Pogue J, Arnold JM et al. Effects of long-term vitamin E supplementation on cardiovascular events and cancer: a randomized controlled trial. *JAMA* 2005; 293(11):1338-1347.

[151] Lonn E, Yusuf S, Hoogwerf B, Pogue J, Yi Q, Zinman B et al. Effects of vitamin E on cardiovascular and microvascular outcomes in high-risk patients with diabetes: results of the HOPE study and MICRO-HOPE substudy. *Diabetes Care* 2002; 25(11):1919-1927.

[152] Kritchevsky SB, Tell GS, Shimakawa T, Dennis B, Li R, Kohlmeier L et al. Provitamin A carotenoid intake and carotid artery plaques: the Atherosclerosis Risk in Communities Study. *Am J Clin Nutr* 1998; 68(3):726-733.

[153] Kushi LH, Folsom AR, Prineas RJ, Mink PJ, Wu Y, Bostick RM. Dietary antioxidant vitamins and death from coronary heart disease in postmenopausal women. *N Engl J Med* 1996; 334(18):1156-1162.

[154] Rimm EB, Stampfer MJ, Ascherio A, Giovannucci E, Colditz GA, Willett WC. Vitamin E consumption and the risk of coronary heart disease in men. *N Engl J Med* 1993; 328(20):1450-1456.

[155] Stampfer MJ, Hennekens CH, Manson JE, Colditz GA, Rosner B, Willett WC. Vitamin E consumption and the risk of coronary disease in women. *N Engl J Med* 1993; 328(20):1444-1449.

[156] Yusuf S, Dagenais G, Pogue J, Bosch J, Sleight P. Vitamin E supplementation and cardiovascular events in high-risk patients. The Heart Outcomes Prevention Evaluation Study Investigators. *N Engl J Med* 2000; 342(3):154-160.

[157] Sesso HD, Buring JE, Norkus EP, Gaziano JM. Plasma lycopene, other carotenoids, and retinol and the risk of cardiovascular disease in men. *Am J Clin Nutr* 2005; 81(5):990-997.

[158] Sesso HD, Buring JE, Norkus EP, Gaziano JM. Plasma lycopene, other carotenoids, and retinol and the risk of cardiovascular disease in women. *Am J Clin Nutr* 2004; 79(1):47-53.

[159] Sesso HD, Liu S, Gaziano JM, Buring JE. Dietary lycopene, tomato-based food products and cardiovascular disease in women. *J Nutr* 2003; 133(7):2336-2341.

[160] Boushey CJ, Beresford SA, Omenn GS, Motulsky AG. A quantitative assessment of plasma homocysteine as a risk factor for vascular disease. Probable benefits of increasing folic acid intakes. *JAMA* 1995; 274(13):1049-1057.

[161] Folsom AR, Nieto FJ, McGovern PG, Tsai MY, Malinow MR, Eckfeldt JH et al. Prospective study of coronary heart disease incidence in relation to fasting total homocysteine, related genetic polymorphisms, and B vitamins: the Atherosclerosis Risk in Communities (ARIC) study. *Circulation* 1998; 98(3):204-210.

[162] Danesh J, Lewington S. Plasma homocysteine and coronary heart disease: systematic review of published epidemiological studies. *J Cardiovasc Risk* 1998; 5(4):229-232.

[163] Ubbink JB, Vermaak WJ, van der MA, Becker PJ. Vitamin B-12, vitamin B-6, and folate nutritional status in men with hyperhomocysteinemia. *Am J Clin Nutr* 1993; 57(1):47-53.

[164] Spoelstra-DE Man AM, Smulders YM, Dekker JM, Heine RJ, Bouter LM, Nijpels G et al. Homocysteine levels are not associated with cardiovascular autonomic function in elderly Caucasian subjects without or with type 2 diabetes mellitus: the Hoorn Study. *J Intern Med* 2005; 258(6):536-543.

[165] Sagara M, Kanda T, NJelekera M, Teramoto T, Armitage L, Birt N et al. Effects of dietary intake of soy protein and isoflavones on cardiovascular disease risk factors in high risk, middle-aged men in Scotland. *J Am Coll Nutr* 2004; 23(1):85-91.

[166] Anderson JW, Johnstone BM, Cook-Newell ME. Meta-analysis of the effects of soy protein intake on serum lipids. *N Engl J Med* 1995; 333(5):276-282.

[167] Wong WW, Smith EO, Stuff JE, Hachey DL, Heird WC, Pownell HJ. Cholesterol-lowering effect of soy protein in normocholesterolemic and hypercholesterolemic men. *Am J Clin Nutr* 1998; 68(6 Suppl):1385S-1389S.

[168] Crouse JR, III, Morgan T, Terry JG, Ellis J, Vitolins M, Burke GL. A randomized trial comparing the effect of casein with that of soy protein containing varying amounts of isoflavones on plasma concentrations of lipids and lipoproteins. *Arch Intern Med* 1999; 159(17):2070-2076.

[169] Teixeira SR, Potter SM, Weigel R, Hannum S, Erdman JW, Jr., Hasler CM. Effects of feeding 4 levels of soy protein for 3 and 6 wk on blood lipids and apolipoproteins in moderately hypercholesterolemic men. *Am J Clin Nutr* 2000; 71(5):1077-1084.

[170] Jenkins DJ, Kendall CW, Mehling CC, Parker T, Rao AV, Agarwal S et al. Combined effect of vegetable protein (soy) and soluble fiber added to a standard cholesterol-lowering diet. *Metabolism* 1999; 48(6):809-816.

[171] Duane WC. Effects of soybean protein and very low dietary cholesterol on serum lipids, biliary lipids, and fecal sterols in humans. *Metabolism* 1999; 48(4):489-494.

[172] Ashton EL, Dalais FS, Ball MJ. Effect of meat replacement by tofu on CHD risk factors including copper induced LDL oxidation. *J Am Coll Nutr* 2000; 19(6):761-767.

[173] Sacks FM, Lichtenstein A, Van Horn L, Harris W, Kris-Etherton P, Winston M. Soy Protein, Isoflavones, and Cardiovascular Health. An American Heart Association Science Advisory for Professionals From the Nutrition Committee. *Circulation* 2006.

[174] Jenkins DJ, Kendall CW, Vuksan V, Vidgen E, Parker T, Faulkner D et al. Soluble fiber intake at a dose approved by the US Food and Drug Administration for a claim of health benefits: serum lipid risk factors for cardiovascular disease assessed in a randomized controlled crossover trial. *Am J Clin Nutr* 2002; 75(5):834-839.

[175] Ziai SA, Larijani B, Akhoondzadeh S, Fakhrzadeh H, Dastpak A, Bandarian F et al. Psyllium decreased serum glucose and glycosylated hemoglobin significantly in diabetic outpatients. *J Ethnopharmacol* 2005; 102(2):202-207.

[176] Jenkins DJ, Wolever TM, Rao AV, Hegele RA, Mitchell SJ, Ransom TP et al. Effect on blood lipids of very high intakes of fiber in diets low in saturated fat and cholesterol. *N Engl J Med* 1993; 329(1):21-26.

[177] Sierra M, Garcia JJ, Fernandez N, Diez MJ, Calle AP. Therapeutic effects of psyllium in type 2 diabetic patients. *Eur J Clin Nutr* 2002; 56(9):830-842.

[178] Heinemann T, Kullak-Ublick GA, Pietruck B, von Bergmann K. Mechanisms of action of plant sterols on inhibition of cholesterol absorption. Comparison of sitosterol and sitostanol. *Eur J Clin Pharmacol* 1991; 40 Suppl 1:S59-S63.

[179] Plat J, Mensink RP. Plant stanol and sterol esters in the control of blood cholesterol levels: mechanism and safety aspects. *Am J Cardiol* 2005; 96(1A):15D-22D.

[180] Grundy SM. Stanol esters as a component of maximal dietary therapy in the National Cholesterol Education Program Adult Treatment Panel III report. *Am J Cardiol* 2005; 96(1A):47D-50D.

[181] Katan MB, Grundy SM, Jones P, Law M, Miettinen T, Paoletti R. Efficacy and safety of plant stanols and sterols in the management of blood cholesterol levels. *Mayo Clin Proc* 2003; 78(8):965-978.

[182] Miettinen TA, Puska P, Gylling H, Vanhanen H, Vartiainen E. Reduction of serum cholesterol with sitostanol-ester margarine in a mildly hypercholesterolemic population. *N Engl J Med* 1995; 333(20):1308-1312.

[183] Gylling H, Miettinen TA. Serum cholesterol and cholesterol and lipoprotein metabolism in hypercholesterolaemic NIDDM patients before and during sitostanol ester-margarine treatment. *Diabetologia* 1994; 37(8):773-780.

[184] Patch CS, Tapsell LC, Williams PG. Plant sterol/stanol prescription is an effective treatment strategy for managing hypercholesterolemia in outpatient clinical practice. *J Am Diet Assoc* 2005; 105(1):46-52.

[185] Cater NB, Garcia-Garcia AB, Vega GL, Grundy SM. Responsiveness of plasma lipids and lipoproteins to plant stanol esters. *Am J Cardiol* 2005; 96(1A):23D-28D.

[186] Jenkins DJ, Kendall CW, Marchie A, Faulkner DA, Wong JM, de Souza R et al. Direct comparison of a dietary portfolio of cholesterol-lowering foods with a statin in hypercholesterolemic participants. *Am J Clin Nutr* 2005; 81(2):380-387.

[187] Salen P, de Lorgeril M. GISSI-Prevenzione trial. *Lancet* 1999; 354(9189):1555-1557.

[188] Matthan NR, Jordan H, Chung M, Lichtenstein AH, Lathrop DA, Lau J. A systematic review and meta-analysis of the impact of omega-3 fatty acids on selected arrhythmia outcomes in animal models. *Metabolism* 2005; 54(12):1557-1565.

[189] Marchioli R, Barzi F, Bomba E, Chieffo C, Di Gregorio D, Di Mascio R et al. Early protection against sudden death by n-3 polyunsaturated fatty acids after myocardial infarction: time-course analysis of the results of the Gruppo Italiano per lo Studio della Sopravvivenza nell'Infarto Miocardico (GISSI)-Prevenzione. *Circulation* 2002; 105(16):1897-1903.

[190] Kris-Etherton PM, Harris WS, Appel LJ. Fish consumption, fish oil, omega-3 fatty acids, and cardiovascular disease. *Circulation* 2002; 106(21):2747-2757.

[191] Burr ML, Fehily AM, Gilbert JF, Rogers S, Holliday RM, Sweetnam PM et al. Effects of changes in fat, fish, and fibre intakes on death and myocardial reinfarction: diet and reinfarction trial (DART). *Lancet* 1989; 2(8666):757-761.

[192] Raitt MH, Connor WE, Morris C, Kron J, Halperin B, Chugh SS et al. Fish oil supplementation and risk of ventricular tachycardia and ventricular fibrillation in patients with implantable defibrillators: a randomized controlled trial. *JAMA* 2005; 293(23):2884-2891.

[193] Brouwer IA, Zock PL, Wever EF, Hauer RN, Camm AJ, Bocker D et al. Rationale and design of a randomised controlled clinical trial on supplemental intake of n-3 fatty acids and incidence of cardiac arrhythmia: SOFA. *Eur J Clin Nutr* 2003; 57(10):1323-1330.

[194] Christensen JH, Riahi S, Schmidt EB, Molgaard H, Kirstein PA, Heath F et al. n-3 Fatty acids and ventricular arrhythmias in patients with ischaemic heart disease and implantable cardioverter defibrillators. *Europace* 2005; 7(4):338-344.

[195] Connor WE. Importance of n-3 fatty acids in health and disease. *Am J Clin Nutr* 2000; 71(1 Suppl):171S-175S.

[196] Harris WS. n-3 fatty acids and serum lipoproteins: human studies. *Am J Clin Nutr* 1997; 65(5 Suppl):1645S-1654S.

INDEX

A

B

C

D

E

F

G

H

I

J

K

L

M

Q

R

S

T

U

V

W

Y

Z